The Arthritis Miracle

The
Arthritis
Miracle

How Ginger Extract Can
Reduce Inflammatory
Joint Pain

Earl Mindell,
R.Ph., Ph.D.

Avery • *a member of*
Penguin Putnam Inc.
New York

The information contained in this book is based upon the research and personal and professional experience of the author. It is not intended as a substitute for consulting with your physician or other health-care provider. Any attempt to diagnose and treat an illness or condition should be done under the direction of a health-care professional.

The publisher and author are not responsible for any adverse effects or consequences resulting from the use of any of the suggestions, preparations, or procedures discussed in this book. Should the reader have any questions concerning the appropriateness of any procedure or preparation method, the author and the publisher strongly suggest consulting a professional health-care adviser.

Most Avery books are available at special quantity discounts for bulk purchase for sales promotions, premiums, fund-raising, and educational needs. Special books or book excerpts also can be created to fit specific needs. For details, write Putnam Special Markets, 375 Hudson Street, New York, NY 10014.

Avery
a member of
Penguin Putnam Inc.
375 Hudson Street
New York, NY 10014
www.penguinputnam.com

Library of Congress Cataloging-in-Publication Data
Mindell, Earl.
    The arthritis miracle : how ginger extract can reduce
inflammatory joint pain / Earl Mindell.
        p.   cm.
    Includes bibliographical references and index.
    ISBN 1-58333-059-3
    1. Arthritis—Alternative treatment.   2. Ginger—Therapeutic use.
I. Title.
    RC933.M565   2000   99–052046
    616.7'2206—dc21

Printed in the United States of America

10   9   8   7   6   5   4   3   2

This book is printed on acid-free paper. ∞

Book design by Jennifer Ann Daddio
Cover designer: Oscar Maldonado
In-house editor: Marie Caratozzolo

Contents

✳

The Arthritis Miracle

Introduction

✳

Arthritis has reached epidemic proportions in developed nations. Approximately 80 million people worldwide suffer from chronic pain and inflammation in their joints, and this number continues to increase. In their search for relief, arthritis sufferers typically use over-the-counter and prescription medications. Some may visit physical therapists for costly treatments that only temporarily relieve discomfort. Others with severe cases may opt to undergo surgery, while still others simply choose to bear the pain. A few natural products have helped alleviate some of the painful symptoms of arthritis, but they vary widely in their effectiveness.

Modern medicine has not yet found a cure for arthritis, and through the process of trying to find one, it has created an entirely new set of problems. Each year, an estimated 100,000 people are hospitalized and 16,000 patients die from side effects caused by commonly prescribed arthritis medications. The need for safer treatment methods has inspired an ongoing flurry of research and drug development by pharmaceutical companies. Recently, new arthritis medications that are touted as having minimal side effects are becoming available through the FDA's "fast-track" approval process. It remains to be seen, however, if these "miracles of science" have long-term effectiveness.

I have been researching nutritional science for thirty years, and I have watched the arthritis problem become more and more serious. I've seen natural remedies for this disease come and go. It wasn't until I met Danish biochemist Dr. Morton Weidner that I believed any of these remedies had the potential to replace the drugs used to treat arthritis pain and inflammation. Dr. Weidner has developed a patented extract from specific subspecies of ginger. This extract is proving to be enormously helpful to arthritis sufferers around the world.

Despite what I had already known of ginger's anti-inflammatory effects, at first I was skeptical of Dr. Weidner's claims, which sounded too good to be true. When I looked through his research and clinical data, however, I became convinced that this patented ginger extract was a major breakthrough in treating arthritis and other inflammatory joint conditions. As positive feedback on this product from arthritis sufferers worldwide began pouring in, it became apparent that this ginger extract has all the potency of a prescription drug for alleviating the painful symptoms of arthritis without the harmful side effects—a perfect meeting of pharmaceutical science and nature. I discovered there was a growing number of arthritis sufferers in the United States, Europe, Asia, and Australia who were using this extract and enjoying relief from their joint pain without any side effects.

In the pages of *The Arthritis Miracle,* you'll learn everything you need to know about arthritis and the drugs commonly used to treat it. You'll also discover the use of ginger—specifically, a ginger extract—to alleviate pain and inflammation.

The book's opening chapter, "The Arthritis Epidemic," provides basic information on arthritis—what it is, how it develops, and the lifestyle changes that can help keep its painful symptoms to a minimum. As it is important to understand the actual causes of inflammation, the next chapter, "Inflammation and Eicosanoids," presents the process that causes joints to ache and swell. Non-steroidal anti-inflammatory drugs and COX-2 inhibitors—the latest drugs prescribed for alleviating arthritis pain—are discussed in yet another chapter. The drawbacks of these and other common drugs prescribed for arthritis also are discussed here.

Subsequent chapters focus on the marvelous healing attributes of ginger, specifically its role in inflammatory joint conditions. "Ginger's Rich Tradition" begins with the illustrious history of this gift of nature that has been used for centuries as both a popular spice and an herbal healer. "Nature's Anti-Inflammatory" details ginger's specific role in reducing inflammation. In this chapter, you will learn why ginger is the superior choice over prescription and over-the-counter medications for the treatment of arthritis, migraine headaches, menstrual cramps, and other inflammatory conditions. Scientific studies supporting the research of ginger extract for relieving arthritis pain and inflammation also are presented. Finally, the links between ginger, a healthy gastrointestinal system, and joint health are discussed in the final chapter.

I have tried to keep the complicated scientific jargon to a minimum. Any terminology you might not be familiar with usually will be italicized and defined. A glossary beginning on page 79 is also provided.

If you have given up hope that you will ever be free from arthritis pain without the help of drugs, you're in for a pleasant surprise. With healthy lifestyle choices and ginger extract—nature's anti-inflammatory—you can ease the pain of inflammatory joint conditions naturally.

Earl Mindell, R.Ph., Ph.D.
Beverly Hills, California

The Arthritis Epidemic

✳

Arthritis is the most common chronic disease in developed nations, affecting some 80 million people worldwide. It can take a number of forms and can affect any joint in the body. General symptoms of arthritis, which include joint stiffness, pain, and inflammation, can range from mild and manageable to severe and unbearable. About 43 million of those afflicted with arthritis are Americans—of which approximately 40 million have osteoarthritis, the most common form of this disease. The remaining 3 million suffer from rheumatoid arthritis. Both forms will be discussed later in this chapter. An estimated 39 million doctor's visits each year are attributed to arthritis.

Degenerative joint diseases are not new. Remains of prehistoric humans and animals show signs of arthritic changes in the joints. Such changes probably were due simply to wear and tear. Today, the increasing numbers of people in westernized countries who are debilitated by arthritis indicate that other factors, such as poor dietary choices, lack of exercise, and the use of certain prescription drugs, may be significant contributors to this epidemic. All of these factors affect the body's biochemical balance, and when this balance is disrupted, the odds of developing arthritis increase. Once the disease sets in, this imbalance accelerates its course. In the next chapter, "Inflammation and Eicosanoids," you'll learn more about this biochemical imbalance. You'll also discover that the typical drug treatments for joint inflammation are only stopgap treatment measures. Although they may temporarily alleviate painful symptoms, they can actually hamper the body's efforts to heal. Ginger extract, as you will see, is the superior choice for correcting these imbalances.

Before discussing the different types of arthritis and other kinds of inflammatory joint and muscle diseases, such as bursitis, tendinitis, gout, carpal tunnel syndrome, and fibromyalgia, let's take a look at how joints work.

How Joints Work

Two types of joints can be affected by arthritis—synovial and cartilaginous. Both types contain a considerable amount of cartilage, which deteriorates in arthritis. *Cartilage* is a layer of dense connective tissue that cushions joints, decreasing friction between bones. It is built around tightly wound strands of protein called *collagen*.

Specialized cells called *chondroblasts* secrete a matrix of carbohydrate and protein molecules into the grid formed by collagen fibers. Smooth, firm, and flexible, cartilage contains no blood vessels but is nourished by the fluids that bathe the joints. These fluids move through the cartilage when the joint is moved. Without this regular nutrient bath, cartilage deteriorates.

Synovial joints include the major joints of the arms and legs. The inner surface of this type of joint is lined with a membrane that produces *hyaluronic acid,* a lubricating fluid. *Synovial fluid* allows the head of the bone to move freely in the socket. Synovial joints also contain cartilage that cushions and lubricates joint movement. *Cartilaginous joints* include the joints between the vertebrae. Between most of the vertebrae of the spine, round cushions of cartilage—often called *discs*—prevent the contact of bone with bone and give the spine its amazing range of movement.

Cartilage isn't the only part of the joint that is damaged by arthritis. The synovial lining, muscles, tendons, ligaments, and even the bones can suffer permanent damage from the chronic inflammation of arthritis.

Osteoarthritis

Osteoarthritis, the most common form of arthritis, affects an estimated 10 percent of the population worldwide. Believed to be caused primarily by wear and tear, osteoarthritis typically affects weight-bearing joints, such as those of the hips, knees, and spine. And because the hands are in constant use, the finger joints are often affected as well. Almost 80 percent of people over age fifty have some degree of osteoarthritis.

Generally osteoarthritis, also known as *degenerative arthritis,* is considered a disease of aging. In it, the spongy, flexible cartilage that cushions areas where bone meets bone begins to wear. As a result, the surfaces within the joint no longer slide over one another smoothly. Once like the perfectly matched pieces of a jigsaw puzzle, the roughened joint surfaces begin to rasp against one another. In cases of advanced osteoarthritis, the body summons its healing forces to try to repair the joint, resulting in a process known as *inflammation.* You'll read about inflammation in Chapter 2, and you'll see how the body's efforts to heal itself can go terribly wrong.

At first, arthritis pain strikes only when the affected joint is being used, but after a while, the joint starts to hurt constantly. As the cartilage wears away, the body tries to repair the joint by building new bone and cartilage. If, however, these structures are not aligned properly, painful bone spurs that reduce range of motion may result.

There are actually several types of osteoarthritis. Fibromyalgia, bursitis, tendinitis, and carpal tunnel syndrome are the most common forms.

- **Bursitis** is painful swelling of the bursae—small sacs found in the connective tissue, usually near joints. These sacs are filled with synovial fluid, which reduces friction between tendons and bones or ligaments. Often, bursitis is the result of prolonged stress or pressure that causes the bursae to become inflamed or swollen. Once inflamed, the swollen sacs press against a neighboring joint, creating pain.

- **Tendinitis** is painful swelling of a tendon—fibrous tissue that attaches muscle to bone. Usually this inflammation is caused by overexertion in sports or other physical activity. Tendinitis commonly occurs in the tendons found in the knee, elbow, and rotator cuff, which stabilizes the shoulder. The Achilles tendon, located at the back of the ankle, also is commonly affected.
- **Carpal tunnel syndrome** is a condition resulting from excessive or repetitive pressure on the median nerve, located in the hand. The median nerve, which controls some of the hand and finger muscles, passes through a tiny opening located below the wrist called the carpal tunnel. Repetitious movement involving the wrist and fingers creates irritation and swelling, which causes the tissue of the carpal tunnel to press on the median nerve. Tingling, numbness, and pain are common symptoms. The repetitive finger motion caused by constantly typing on a computer keyboard or punching keys on a cash register can cause carpal tunnel syndrome.
- **Fibromyalgia** is a disorder that is characterized by muscle and joint pain that persists for no apparent

reason. The cause of this condition, which affects about 10 million Americans and is closely associated with chronic fatigue syndrome, is not clearly understood.

In some instances, inherited structural problems, such as joint misalignment, can cause individuals to be prone to arthritis. Such misalignments cause the cartilage to wear down easily. Those with such a predisposition should take preventive measures against osteoarthritis, including regular strengthening and stretching exercises, proper diet, and attention to good posture—preferably under the guidance of a physical therapist.

Others who may be prone to arthritis are those whose occupations demand sitting in chairs or vehicles for much of the day. Years of this type of posture, coupled with lack of proper exercise, commonly causes the hips and spine to become misaligned. In turn, the joints in the legs and neck also are knocked out of proper alignment, resulting in stress on the cartilaginous surfaces within the joints.

Repetitive stress on certain joints also increases the risk of osteoarthritis. Athletes, dancers, and those who do repetitive physical labor are at risk of wearing away the cartilage in the joints they use most. But don't think that lying around as a couch potato will protect you from osteoarthritis, either. Those who don't get proper exercise are at increased risk as well. Joints that are not moved regularly through their full range of motion are far more likely to deteriorate with age.

Other known risk factors for osteoarthritis include obesity, smoking, and a family history of the disease. And if you have injured a joint, there is a greater likelihood of that area becoming arthritic.

There is no cure for osteoarthritis. Although cartilage can rebuild itself, there is no surefire way to reverse the process that destroyed it in the first place. Living with chronic pain can be a waking nightmare. Especially painful is arthritis that affects the intervertebral discs of the spine. Muscles tighten and nerves can become entrapped. If you have ever suffered from back pain, you know that when your back hurts, it's hard to function. Each year, back pain is responsible for putting 7 million people temporarily out of work.

Most approaches for arthritis involve controlling the pain and inflammation with drugs and allowing the body to heal itself to the best of its ability. The most common drugs for alleviating the painful symptoms of osteoarthritis include non-steroidal anti-inflammatory drugs (NSAIDs) and steroid drugs like cortisone. Later in this book, you'll learn more about these drugs and their harmful side effects, and you will also see why ginger extract is the superior alternative.

Arthroscopic surgery is another treatment method for relieving friction within arthritic joints. Through this procedure, a tiny catheter is introduced into the joint where it smooths out bumpy cartilage surfaces. In very severe cases, arthritic joints are surgically replaced with artificial ones. Although these procedures have helped many people deal with arthritis, any surgical procedure has inherent risks and is costly. In many cases, they need to be repeated. It also is expensive and risky, and in arthritis cases, should be considered only by those who are crippled by the disease. Many millions simply live with the chronic pain. Osteoarthritis sufferers need other solutions.

Rheumatoid Arthritis

Rheumatoid arthritis (RA), also referred to as *inflammatory arthritis*, is categorized as an autoimmune disorder. In it, the immune system mistakenly attacks the body's own tissues, causing chronic and damaging levels of inflammation, pain, and joint swelling. Joints of the hands, feet, wrists, knees, hips, and ankles most commonly are affected. Rheumatoid arthritis affects three to five times as many women as men, and generally occurs between the ages of twenty and forty.

Initially, a joint's synovial membranes become inflamed, which cause it to swell and become stiff. As a result, the inflamed membranes emit enzymes that break down the joint cartilage. The cartilage is replaced by fibrous tissue, which can calcify and form bony knobs that may fuse the joint, restricting movement.

Let's take a closer look at this process. Within the

joint spaces affected by rheumatoid arthritis, immune cells called *lymphocytes* react to what they think are foreign substances. Lymphocytes are the messengers that summon the troops of the immune system into action, which causes the formation of chemicals called *cytokines.* Cytokines are the "generals" of the immune army; they give orders to other types of immune cells that cause the inflammatory response. In the case of rheumatoid arthritis and other autoimmune diseases, the lymphocytes and cytokines overreact by summoning an entire platoon of immune cells, when all they really need are a few good men. So, instead of simply eradicating the enemy, they start fighting amongst themselves and tearing up the landscape in the process.

What causes this overreaction that ultimately destroys joint tissues? Complementary medical practitioners believe the answer lies mainly in diet. In nations that consume the Western diet, which, in large part, is composed of processed foods that are void of vital nutrients, autoimmune diseases are far more common. Regular diets of these foods coupled with the use of NSAIDs have been linked to a condition known as *leaky gut syndrome,* which is believed to be linked to rheumatoid arthritis.

Leaky gut is actually an erosion of the gastrointestinal tract that results in tiny holes in the intestinal lining. Through this breached intestinal wall, partially digested food particles, bacteria, and other toxic microorganisms are able to pass directly into the bloodstream. Because these "invaders" don't belong in the blood, the immune system is called into action to fight them, resulting in inflammation. Furthermore, some of these toxins, which closely resemble certain joint tissues, make their way to the joints. When the immune system begins its attack, it doesn't discriminate very well and wages its war against the toxins, as well as the healthy joints themselves. One result of this immune reaction is rheumatoid arthritis. When the gut is allowed to heal through a nutritious whole foods, non-allergenic diet, rheumatoid arthritis symptoms improve.

Most people with rheumatoid arthritis have periods of intense inflammation and pain alternating with periods of improved joint health throughout their lives. In 20 percent of the cases, the condition simply disappears and does not return. It usually is treated with NSAIDs, steroids, and immunosuppressive drugs. Physical therapy usually is necessary for those with this condition, and, if the joints are deteriorated badly, replacement surgery may be needed to avoid total disability.

Other Forms of Arthritis

There are a number of other types of arthritis. *Ankylosing spondylitis* is an autoimmune form of this disease in which the joints of the vertebrae become inflamed and rigid. In severe cases, they may fuse together. Ankylosing spondylitis affects more than twice as many men as women.

Gout, an acute form of inflammatory arthritis, typically affects the smaller joints of the feet (especially the big toe) and hands. Joint swelling and pain result from deposits of crystallized uric acid salt. About 90 percent of the 1 million Americans who suffer from gout are males. Typically, those affected are overweight and regularly eat rich foods and drink alcoholic beverages.

Infectious arthritis is caused by a bacterial, viral, or fungal infection. Usually the infectious organism travels through the bloodstream to a joint. An injury or surgery can result in this type of arthritis as well. Redness, swelling, and tenderness, often coupled with fever and body aches, is characteristic of infectious arthritis.

Other disorders such as *Lyme disease* and *lupus* can cause arthritic-like symptoms as well.

Summing It Up

Now that you are aware of the different types of arthritis, in the next chapter, you'll see how diet, stress, and dependence on certain medications can upset the body's inflammatory hormonal balance. You'll also learn how to restore this balance.

Inflammation and Eicosanoids

＊

Inflammation is one way in which the body reacts to injury or illness. Any area of the body—external or internal—can display an *inflammatory response.* External inflammation is generally the result of an injury. Consider, for instance, the *external* inflammatory response in the tissues of a sprained ankle. The area will swell, turn red, and become painful. Common causes of an *internal* inflammatory response include bacterial infections, allergies, and arthritis. During an asthma attack, for example, the air passages are inflamed, making it difficult to breathe. When allergies flare, inflammation may cause a runny nose, watery eyes, and perhaps an outbreak of hives. Inflammatory bowel diseases, including Crohn's disease and ulcerative colitis, are examples of internal inflammation. These conditions are characterized by inflammation of the inner surface of the large intestine, and commonly result in abdominal pain, diarrhea, and bloody stools. A fever is an example of whole body inflammation. And arthritis causes inflammation of the joints, resulting in swelling and pain.

Exactly what happens during the inflammatory process? To illustrate, let's take the example of a sprained ankle. An ankle sprain occurs when one of the tendons that attaches your lower leg muscles to your foot is overstretched abruptly. The sudden shock tears some of the fibers that make up that tendon. Immediately, hormonal messengers called *eicosanoids* send out a message to specialized immune cells to get to the injured area and begin their healing efforts. As immune system cells migrate to the area that's injured, they pull fluid along with them, causing the area to swell. The activity of the tissue repair generates heat and causes redness.

Too much inflammation, however, can cause great harm. In the case of arthritis, uncontrolled inflammation can cause intense fluid pressure within the joint. This pressure, coupled with the free radicals produced during the inflammatory process, can destroy tissues in the area.

Free radicals are atoms or groups of atoms that contain at least one unpaired electron (electrons usually occur in pairs, maintaining chemical stability). When an electron is unpaired, it hooks up easily with another molecule and can cause a harmful chemical reaction. Normally present in the body in small amounts, free radicals are necessary for the production of energy and other metabolic processes. Under normal circumstances, they are neutralized by substances known as *antioxidants*. The trouble occurs when there is excessive free-radical formation. Damage to cells, tissues, and weakness to the immune system eventually can result in a host of degenerative diseases and other health conditions.

Free radicals are caused by a number of factors, including exposure to radiation, and environmental pollutants such as car exhaust, smog, and other environmental pollutants. Diet also contributes to the formation of free radicals. When the body metabolizes nutrients through diet, it utilizes these nutrients along with oxygen to produce energy. During this *oxidation* process, oxygen molecules containing free radicals are released. Again, antioxidants neutralize these free radicals. A high-fat diet can increase free-radical activity because oxidation occurs more readily in fat molecules than it does in carbohydrate or protein molecules.

You could liken free radicals to the exhaust created by the engine of a car. In order to create energy from fuel, cars create hazardous exhaust. In much the same way, the body creates hazardous waste when it burns fuel for energy during metabolism.

When you slice an apple and leave it exposed to the air, oxidation causes it to turn brown. If you add lemon juice to the sliced apple, it will stay crisp and white for a longer period because the vitamin C in the lemon juice acts as an antioxidant. Antioxidants in the body help keep free radicals in check, preventing them from causing significant cell damage. When inflammation is out of control, however, free radicals outnumber antioxidants and begin to destroy cells in the affected area. In addition to dietary antioxidants like vitamin C and vitamin E, there are dozens of other plant-based substances that act as antioxidants in the body—including several of the active ingredients of ginger.

Bodies Out of Balance

Many of our modern medical conditions can be traced back to an inflammatory process that has run amok. Allergies, asthma, osteoarthritis, and rheumatoid arthritis and other autoimmune diseases, such as Crohn's disease, ulcerative colitis, and lupus, all involve inflammation that is out of control. New research is investigating a possible link between the chronic inflammation and the development of heart disease and cancer (see discussion beginning on page 58).

What makes inflammation spiral out of control, causing permanent tissue damage? In the majority of instances, a body out of balance is to blame. Poor diet and chronic stress change the levels of eicosanoids, which are important for controlling inflammation. When the balance of these hormones is thrown off, and inflammation occurs, the body is set to overreact.

Modern medicine's answer for combating excess

inflammation, as it is with just about every other illness, is handed out on pages torn from prescription pads. Non-steroidal anti-inflammatory drugs (NSAIDs), such as ibuprofen, aspirin, and acetaminophen, are commonly prescribed. Steroid drugs, including cortisone (oral and injectable) are prescribed for cases of inflammation that cannot be managed with NSAIDs. You'll see, however, that NSAIDs and steroid drugs cause as many problems as they solve.

The Eicosanoids

Prostaglandins, leukotrienes, and thromboxanes are hormones known as *eicosanoids*. Unlike other kinds of hormones, which travel through the bloodstream from the glands to distant points throughout the body, eicosanoids act locally on the cells that produce them or on other cells in the immediate vicinity. They are created and vanish within a fraction of a second. Each type of eicosanoid carries out its own duties in the body, with a few overlapping functions.

Prostaglandins, so named because they were discovered in the prostate gland, were the first of these elusive hormones to be discovered. Since then, dozens of different eicosanoid hormones have been discovered to work throughout the body. The more we learn about them, the more we learn about what causes chronic illnesses such as arthritis. Nearly every cell in the body makes locally acting hormones, and science is only beginning to unlock their mysteries.

Prostaglandins, leukotrienes, and thromboxanes have different, yet sometimes overlapping job responsibilities in the body. Each eicosanoid has many subtypes. For example, prostaglandin subtypes include prostaglandins B_1, A_3, E_1, E_2, A_2, and B_2. While one prostaglandin subtype may work to constrict blood vessels and increase inflammation, another subtype will prevent these actions from going too far. Each subtype has a different function in the body. To maintain proper balance, the subtypes within each eicosanoid class are involved in a kind of checks and balances system.

Prostaglandins modify the immune system, pain response, inflammation, body temperature, the constriction and expansion of blood vessels, blood clotting, and the health of the stomach lining. Leukotrienes modify inflammation, the immune response, mucus secretion, and muscle contractions. Thromboxanes modify blood clotting and pain sensations.

Balance Is Everything

Balance is everything when it comes to eicosanoids. Overlapping functions of eicosanoids are designed to provide a system of checks and balances. For instance, if a prostaglandin subtype that increases pain sensation is not balanced by another subtype that decreases pain, the painful sensation will worsen. By the same token, if a leukotriene that causes increased inflammation is not balanced by one that turns off the inflammatory response at the appropriate time, then that response can harm healthy tissues.

The best way to understand this balance is to divide eicosanoids into "good" and "bad" categories. The "good" eicosanoids have health-supporting, positive effects. They help do the following:

- decrease inflammation throughout the body.
- maintain the proper consistency of blood, making it less likely to clot.
- improve immune system function.
- expand the walls of blood vessels, lowering blood pressure and improving circulation.
- protect the stomach lining from being burned by stomach acids.
- prevent the multiplication of cancer cells.

The harmful effects of "bad" eicosanoids cause a swing in the opposite direction. They do the following:

- encourage inflammation.
- cause blood to thicken.
- decrease immune system function.
- cause blood vessel walls to constrict.

Keep in mind that all of these hormones are necessary and that when they are in perfect balance, they counteract each other to provide an optimal environment. Problems arise when an imbalance tips the scale toward the pro-inflammatory, vessel-constrictive, blood-thickening, immune-compromising eicosanoids.

To further explain this, take the following example. Prostaglandin E_2 (PGE_2) causes pain and fever. It is one of the principal targets of aspirin and NSAIDs, which inhibit the production of this pro-inflammatory eicosanoid. PGE_2 plays an important role in the development of arthritis and other inflammatory diseases. It also decreases the activity of an immune component that seeks out and kills cancer cells. Because of PGE_2's effects on cancer cells, research into the possible anti-cancer effects of aspirin and NSAIDs is beginning to pick up steam. Because ginger extract works by the same mechanism as NSAIDs, it's possible that it can provide the same anti-cancer effects.

Prostaglandin E_1 (PGE_1), on the other hand, inhibits the clumping of blood components called platelets; it also opens up constricted blood vessels and strengthens the immune system. When PGE_1 and PGE_2 are balanced, inflammation is controlled and blood flows freely through the blood vessels. If PGE_2 is more abundant, its negative effects predominate.

Other types of prostaglandins cause blood vessels to expand and become more permeable, so that their presence at the site of inflammation brings in more fluid. Increased fluid pressure leads to increased pain and tissue damage.

There are certain leukotrienes that increase mucus

secretion, and other leukotrienes that decrease it. Some leukotrienes attract unnecessarily large numbers of immune cells to the area of inflammation, strongly upgrading the inflammatory response. If too many of these leukotrienes are present, inflammation can easily get out of hand.

If there is too much of any one eicosanoid subtype and not enough of another, the body's physiological balance point shifts slightly. It appears that a number of modern lifestyle choices, such as diets of sugar-laden and processed foods, lack of exercise, and high stress levels, shift that point toward inflammation.

The Making of Eicosanoids

Eicosanoids are made from essential fatty acids (EFAs)—polyunsaturated fats that are necessary for optimal health. Because the body is not able to produce EFAs, they must be obtained through the diet. Therefore, the balance of "good" and "bad" eicosanoids in the body is largely determined by the kinds of fatty acids found in the foods you eat. Once fats are digested and the fatty acids pass into the bloodstream, cells throughout the body begin turning them into eicosanoids. Enzymes are the tools that cells use to build eicosanoids of the raw material of fatty acids.

Think of your cells as tiny factories that are capable of making several different products. Which product gets manufactured depends on the raw materials that are available. Say you eat a piece of fresh salmon. During the digestive process, your body liberates the omega-3 fats, one type of EFA, contained in the fish. Omega-3 fats contain alpha-linolenic acid (ALA), which is transformed by the enzymes *delta 6-desaturase* and *delta 5-desaturase* into eicosapentaenoic acid (EPA). EPA is then transformed by *cyclooxygenase (COX) enzymes* into "good" prostaglandins, and by *lipoxygenase* enzymes into "good" leukotrienes.

Omega-3 fats, which are found in fish oils and certain vegetable oils including canola and flaxseed, have positive health effects because they serve as the raw material for "good" eicosanoids only. Specifically, these fats are a part of nutritional treatments for heart disease, inflammatory bowel diseases, high blood pressure, weakness of the immune system, and rheumatoid arthritis. A recommended dosage of 200 milligrams of EPA per day helps to ensure the production of anti-inflammatory, blood-thinning, immune-boosting, and blood vessel-opening eicosanoids.

If, on the other hand, you eat a food that is rich in a polyunsaturated fat like corn oil, omega-6 fats, the other type of EFAs, are released in the body. These fats, which also are found in other vegetable oils, raw nuts, seeds, and legumes, contain linoleic acid. Linoleic acid is transformed into gamma-linoleic acid (GLA) and then to dihomo-gamma-linoleic acid (DHGLA). Now the body comes to a crossroads. The DHGLA can be transformed either into arachidonic acid, from which "bad" eicosanoids are created, or into "good" eicosanoids.

Arachidonic acid is the raw material from which pro-inflammatory eicosanoids are made. It is considered a non-essential fatty acid because it can be produced in the body from omega-6 fats. The Western diet, which typically is high in meat and dairy products, has too much arachidonic acid and omega-6 fats from vegetable oils, and not enough omega-3s. This creates an imbalance between the raw materials for the eicosanoids that control pain and inflammation.

Arachidonic acid from meat and dairy products, as well as from the omega-6 fats, can be made into "good" or "bad" eicosanoids. How does the body decide which type of eicosanoid should be made from arachidonic acid? It depends upon the presence of certain enzymes. When an enzyme called *cyclooxygenase-2* (COX-2) is present, pro-inflammatory prostaglandins are made from arachidonic acid. Inflammatory leukotrienes are formed if the enzyme *5-lipoxygenase* is present. Keep in mind that when 5-lipoxygenase or COX-2 acts on EPA from omega-3 fats, they create good leukotrienes and prostaglandins, but when they act on arachidonic acid, they create harmful pro-inflammatory leukotrienes and prostaglandins.

As you will see in the next chapter, most drugs used to treat arthritis work by inhibiting COX-2 enzymes. Inhibiting COX-2 and 5-lipoxygenase stops inflammation and pain from spinning out of control. Later on, you'll discover how ginger extract also can inhibit these enzymes without any negative side effects.

Think of the eicosanoid pathway as a set of train tracks, and omega-6 fats as the train. Cyclooxygenases and lipoxygenases are conductors. When COX-2 is on the job, it turns the train down the tracks that lead to the production of harmful pro-inflammatory prostaglandins. When lipoxygenase is driving, its route goes to "bad" leukotrienes. The presence of either of these enzymes takes the train to these destinations. (Omega-3s, on the other hand, go on one set of tracks only and cannot veer off course.)

Specifically, what affects eicosanoid balance? Mainly diet and stress levels, which are presented in the following discussions.

Diet and Eicosanoid Balance

In his groundbreaking book *Enter the Zone*, biochemist Barry Sears describes how the foods we eat affect eicosanoid balance. The two enzymes delta 6-desaturase and delta 5-desaturase activate the essential fatty acids. First, delta-6 activates linoleic acid (omega-6) and alpha-linolenic (omega-3) acids. Then delta-5 acts upon these activated fatty acids to create arachidonic acid (from linoleic acid) and eicosapentaenoic acid (from alpha-linolenic acid). If active delta 5-desaturase is not abundantly present, omega-6s are channeled into forming good eicosanoids.

According to Dr. Sears, the activity of delta 5-

desaturase is what determines the direction of the eicosanoid cascade (pathway). If this enzyme is very active, the balance shifts toward the formation of arachidonic acid, and, therefore, toward the production of harmful eicosanoids. So what causes the activity of delta-5? The answer is insulin—the metabolic hormone responsible for balancing blood sugar.

A diet high in refined carbohydrates and sugars and low in protein stimulates insulin production. Through the refining process, foods such as grains and sugarcane are stripped of precious fiber and oils, leaving only the carbohydrate core to be rapidly digested. This causes blood sugar levels to shoot up quickly, which, in turn, causes a surge of insulin in an effort to bring the levels back down. High insulin levels lead to the overproduction of arachidonic acid, which results in the overproduction of harmful eicosanoids. Simply put, refined carbohydrates and sugars overexcite the enzymes responsible for making harmful eicosanoids. The enzymes shift into glucose-powered high gear and churn out the hormones that set the stage for inflammation.

The ideal diet for eicosanoid balance includes plenty of low-fat protein, vegetables, whole grains, and small amounts of fresh fruit. It contains little or no refined sugars or refined grains. For optimum health, try to eat fish at least twice a week, and eliminate as many processed foods from your diet as possible, especially those made with hydrogenated vegetable oils (margarines, vegetable shortening, and many prepared packaged foods), which disrupt the important activity of delta-6. Limit the consumption of red meat. To help balance other fats, include omega-3 rich walnuts and flaxseeds in your diet.

Stress and Eicosanoid Balance

As you have seen, the delta 6-desaturase enzyme is needed to transform linoleic and alpha-linolenic acids into activated fatty acids. This is a crucial step in the synthesis of eicosanoid hormones. When the body is under stress, hormonal changes take place. Specifically, the body pumps out the hormones adrenaline and cortisol. Among other harmful bodily effects, these hormones impede the important activity of delta 6-desaturase and cause increased insulin levels. In other words, being under stress can upset the balance between "good" and "bad" eicosanoids.

Summing It Up

This chapter has given you an idea of the complex systems your body uses to make eicosanoids. You also have seen how hormonal imbalance plays a major role in creating inflammation, including that which is associated with the pain and joint destruction of arthritis.

The pharmaceutical industry is busy trying to create drugs that inhibit this process by affecting eicosanoid balance. Unfortunately, these medicines tend to work like blunt instruments, knocking out whole classes of eicosanoids, which further disrupts hormonal equilibrium in the long run. Ginger extract, on the other hand, works in harmony with the body, selectively dampening the effects of the pro-inflammatory leukotrienes and prostaglandins. In the next chapter, "NSAIDs and the COX Connection," you'll learn about the benefits of commonly prescribed anti-inflammatory drugs as well as their serious downside.

3

NSAIDs and the COX Connection

✳

Hugh was a high-powered publishing company executive. He worked long days and enjoyed the constant challenges of his career. He had no intention of retiring, despite the fact that he was about to celebrate his sixty-fifth birthday. He thrived on the high-stress, fast-paced atmosphere of publishing.

An avid tennis player, Hugh gradually started developing painful osteoarthritis in both knees. At first, he took Advil daily to stave off the pain, but eventually this over-the-counter medication stopped doing the job. His doctor assured him not to worry, and prescribed daily doses of indomethacin (Indocin), a stronger prescription non-steroidal anti-inflammatory drug (NSAID). He told Hugh that he could probably continue to play tennis and live relatively pain-free. After a few months on Indocin, Hugh's knees felt pretty good and hurt only when he overdid it on the tennis court. He began to notice, however, a worrisome burning sensation in his stomach.

When the doctor heard of Hugh's stomach problems, he explained that sometimes indomethacin irritated the stomach and could cause ulcers. In an attempt to prevent any stomach problems, he put Hugh on an acid-suppressing drug called cimetidine (Tagamet). Hugh dutifully took his medications, but his general health began to deteriorate over the next several months. His skin became dry and prone to rashes, he was always tired and listless, and it seemed as if he was always fighting a cold or the flu. Although Hugh never had allergies, he began to develop sensitivities to pollen, as well as to his two beloved golden retrievers. His doctor added an antihistamine and a muscle relaxant to his growing list of medications. When his stomach began to burn uncomfortably again, the doctor recommended that Hugh add Tums to his daily regimen.

Soon, Hugh found that he could no longer stay focused enough to do his job. Reluctantly, he decided to retire. He had always imagined that his retirement would mean lots of time for his favorite sports, travel, and volunteer work. He found, however, that he had only enough energy for sitting in his easy chair and watching television. He became depressed and eventually ended up with a prescription for the antidepressant Prozac on top of all the other medications he was taking. It was becoming difficult to keep track of them all.

One evening, Hugh felt particularly sick. The pains in his stomach seemed stronger than usual. His wife took him to the local hospital emergency room. Tests revealed that Hugh was suffering from serious internal bleeding. The doctor who took care of him at the hospital told Hugh that if he hadn't come in that night, he probably would have died in his sleep.

The Arthritis Drug Treadmill

We've been led to believe that over-the-counter pain-killers like ibuprofen (Advil), ketoprofen (Orudis), aspirin, and naproxen (Aleve) are safe to use as often as we like. (See the list on page 36 for a listing of commonly used NSAIDs.) Many people take them daily for headaches, muscle aches, and arthritis pain. The truth is that these and stronger prescription NSAIDs may be effective in decreasing inflammation and pain, but at great cost. These medications typically cause gastrointestinal side effects, such as ulcers, nausea, and stomach discomfort and pain. Individuals with rheumatoid arthritis who use NSAIDs are six and a half times more likely to experience gastrointestinal problems than those with the disease who don't use these drugs. Each year, 7,600 Americans actually die from the side effects of NSAIDs, usually as the result of bleeding ulcers.

What happened to Hugh is far from unusual. He's one of the millions of youthful, energetic people who climb onto the arthritis drug treadmill, convinced that prescription drugs are the only way to find pain relief. They begin with an anti-inflammatory drug to ease arthritis pain. When this medication begins irritating their gastrointestinal tracts, they get another prescription, this time for a stomach acid-reducing medication. When these drugs suppress stomach acid, digestion isn't complete and nutrients aren't absorbed efficiently. As detailed in Chapter 6, this can result in low-level malnutrition, lack of energy, allergy development, and a depressed immune system. What usually follows next are prescriptions for antihistamines and/or antidepressants. Climbing onto the arthritis drug treadmill can be the beginning of a serious decline in health for people over age sixty-five. The elderly are at the greatest risk for gastrointestinal side effects, because their bodies don't metabolize medications as well as they did in their youth. It's alarming to consider how many people in relatively good health—with the exception of painful joints—have ended up in nursing homes because of this downward spiral of increasing medication use.

Even though some people don't experience gastrointestinal problems with NSAIDs, these drugs have other side effects that can compromise quality of life. This is especially true for arthritis sufferers who take them every day. Liver and kidney damage, rashes, dizziness, ringing in the ears, and itchy skin are other common complaints from NSAID users.

Besides all of this, although NSAIDs may decrease inflammation, they also inhibit the formation of cartilage in the joints. They interfere with the synthesis of collagen, the building block of cartilage. Millions of people with deteriorating cartilage take prescription drugs that rob their bodies of the ability to rebuild it.

Arthritis sufferers who have had to stop using NSAIDs often treat their pain with acetaminophen (Tylenol), which works differently from the other NSAIDs. Rather than inhibit COX enzymes, acetaminophen blocks pain impulses in the nervous system. The good news is that it eases pain without causing ulcers or gastrointestinal bleeding. The problem, however, is that it doesn't do anything to control inflammation. And if inflammation isn't controlled in arthritis, joint damage is much more likely to occur. If your joints are inflamed but don't hurt, it's far more likely that you'll injure them further. Why? Because you won't get the pain signals warning you to back off. Acetaminophen also can be dangerous to the liver, especially if too much is used or if it's taken with alcohol.

Commonly Used NSAIDs

aspirin

choline magnesium trisalicylate (Trilisate)

diclofenac (Cataflam, Voltaren, Arthrotec)

diflunisal (Dolobid)

etodolac (Lodine)

fenoprofen (Nalfon)

flurbiprofen (Ansaid)

ibuprofen (Advil)

indomethacin (Indocin)

ketoprofen (Oruvail)

magnesium salicylate (Magan)

meclofenamate (Meclomen)

misoprostol (Arthrotec)

nabumetone (Relafen)

naproxen (Aleve, Anaprox, Naprosyn-EC, Naprelan, Naprosyn)

oxaprozin (Daypro)

piroxicam (Feldene)

salsalate (Disalcid, Salflex, Mono-Gesic)

sulindac (Clinoril)

tolmetin (Tolectin)

twelve-hour aspirin (Zorprin)

The COX-2 Connection

NSAIDs reduce inflammation by decreasing the production of pro-inflammatory prostaglandins. They do this by inhibiting the cyclooxygenase (COX) enzymes. As discussed in the previous chapter, COX enzymes are needed for the formation of both "good" prostaglandins (from omega-3 fats) and "bad" prostaglandins (from omega-6 fats).

Aspirin—the original NSAID—was used for decades before anyone knew how it worked. In 1971, British researcher John Vane was awarded the Nobel Prize for discovering that aspirin relieved inflammation and pain by inhibiting the action of COX enzymes. Since then, other drugs have been designed to have the same action, thus stopping the production of bad eicosanoids. Unfortunately, the action of NSAIDs is analogous to poisoning the whole garden to kill off a single weed. The inhibition of COX enzymes ended up causing untoward side effects because not all COX enzymes produce bad eicosanoids. Some help produce good ones as well.

In the early 1990s, researchers discovered that COX enzymes fall into two categories—COX-1 and COX-2. COX-1 enzymes are needed for the manufacture of prostaglandins that protect the stomach lining and kidneys, while COX-2 enzymes are needed to make harmful pro-inflammatory prostaglandins. Most NSAIDs inhibit *both* types of COX enzymes. In other words, dampening the inflammatory fire of arthritis means leaving the stomach lining and kidneys vulnerable to damage.

Since the discovery of these two different types of COX enzymes, researchers have found that COX-2 may play a role in causing other types of pain, Alzheimer's disease, colon cancer, kidney disease, and osteoporosis. Knowing what you know now about eicosanoids and the many roles they play in the body, you can see that this makes sense. Eicosanoids out of balance have widespread effects.

The Hype Over COX-2 Inhibitors

Drug companies have developed new NSAIDs that *selectively inhibit* COX-2 enzymes. These COX-2 inhibitors, including meloxicam, celecoxib, and rofecoxib, are designed to prevent the formation of pro-inflammatory prostaglandins without gastrointestinal side effects.

In its first few months on the market, celecoxib (Celebrex) became a blockbuster moneymaker for the pharmaceutical company Searle, a subsidiary of Monsanto Company. In its first week on the market, Celebrex was prescribed to 9,923 Americans. Within thirteen weeks, it had been prescribed to 2.5 million arthritis sufferers in the United States alone. (To put this in perspective, know that Viagra, the hugely popular drug for male impotence, sold 2.7 million prescriptions in the same amount of time.) Celebrex is also being considered by the FDA for the treatment of a wider variety of conditions related to pain and inflammation.

Rofecoxib (Vioxx) has been approved for use against arthritis pain as well. Additional studies are looking at Vioxx as a treatment for pain after surgery, menstrual cramps, and tooth pain. There is some dispute over whether meloxicam preferentially inhibits COX-2. The other drugs in this class inhibit COX-2 much more effectively.

While these drugs are a step up from the original NSAIDs, they may not live up to all of the hype that has been created about them. Why? The FDA has sent drug manufacturers, physicians, pharmacists, and the public a clear message that many more long-term studies are needed to determine whether these "super aspirins" are indeed safer than traditional NSAIDs. Pharmaceutical companies are required to label COX-2 inhibitors with a warning about possible adverse gastrointestinal effects. The label informs patients that they have a 1 percent chance of developing ulcers or internal bleeding within the first three to six months of treatment, and 2 to 4 percent after a year. Users are also warned that ulcers caused by these drugs, specifically Celebrex, often crop up without any warning, so they are advised to keep an eye out for signs of gastrointestinal bleeding.

While this may not sound significant, consider the huge numbers of people taking these drugs. According to these figures, if the 2.5 million people who were prescribed celecoxib take it for a year, 50,000 to 100,000 of these users can expect to have serious gastrointestinal side effects.

On April 20, 1999, an article in the *Wall Street Journal* reported that Celebrex had been linked to eleven cases of gastrointestinal hemorrhage and ten deaths (half of which were due to gastrointestinal hemorrhage). Searle's vice president in charge of arthritis research responded to the article by stating that the drug was "performing as expected," and that many patients who experienced side effects from Celebrex had other illnesses and had been taking other drugs—any of which could have caused their negative reactions.

These super aspirin medications are also very expensive—at the time of this writing, they cost approximately three dollars per dose. And like any prescription drug, they carry the risk of harmful interactions with other drugs. Asthmatics and those with high blood pressure or heart conditions are at increased health risk when using COX-2 inhibitors.

Why, if these new NSAIDs affect only COX-2 enzymes, leaving the COX-1 types alone to continue making "good" eicosanoids, do these side effects still occur? For one thing, the function of the COX enzymes isn't totally specific. COX-1 and COX-2 have overlapping functions, and neither is responsible for the creation of only "good" or "bad" prostaglandins. It appears that COX-2 plays a role in tissue repair and in maintaining proper blood flow through the kidneys. Blood flow through the kidneys is an important barometer for the body, helping it regulate proper blood pressure.

Research also indicates that users of Celebrex may be increasing their risk of heart attack and stroke dramatically. It appears that this drug may be implicated in suppressing the body's formation of a prostaglandin called *prostacyclin,* which thins the blood and dilates the blood vessels.

Targeting potent pharmaceuticals at such a specific action in the body is usually a setup for trouble, because the body is rarely that specific itself. The "magic bullet" of drug therapy usually doesn't hit exactly on target. Even when it does, it generally turns out that the target isn't completely responsible for causing the disease being treated. This is why nearly all drugs have adverse effects.

Summing It Up

NSAIDs, while helpful to some degree in alleviating the pain of arthritis, certainly have their share of side effects. Even the latest "super aspirins," which are designed to target only the COX-2 enzymes, may have their drawbacks. In the following chapters, you'll discover that ginger extract is the safe, effective answer. It relieves arthritis pain and inflammation without causing any negative side effects or dangerous interactions with other drugs.

4

Ginger's Rich Tradition

✳

Of all the remedies in the herbalist's medicine cabinet, ginger has the longest and most colorful history. It has graced the tables of people all over the world as a spice and has been used for centuries as a healing agent. The earliest records of ginger are over five thousand years old. Since 200 BC this gift of nature has been used as both a culinary herb and an herbal remedy for a wide spectrum of ills. Historians have discovered records dating back to the fourth century BC that list many of the medical conditions treated by ginger. As a spice, ginger is a mainstay in the traditional foods of China, Japan, and other Asian countries, and its popularity has spread through many countries throughout the world. Gingerbread men and houses, as well as ginger ale and ginger snaps, are traditional parts of folktales and seasonal celebrations.

By the ninth century AD, ginger was imported to

Europe. (It could not be cultivated there because of the climate.) For many centuries, it was used there only by the wealthy. The writings of explorers Marco Polo and Vasco da Gama mention their first experiences of this exotic spice. Nations fought over trade routes for ginger, knowing that control of this wildly popular flavoring would mean riches. The thirteenth through sixteenth centuries witnessed ginger's introduction in East Africa, Malaysia, the West Indies, and parts of Africa.

Ginger is included in ancient Arab religious texts and folklore and is still a part of some religious rituals of that culture. In the early twentieth century, anthropologists reported that natives of Papua, New Guinea, ritually spat ginger onto the roads leading into their villages for good luck. It has also been found in centuries-old tombs of Chinese monarchy, and its aphrodisiac effects are highlighted in *The Arabian Nights*. Several works of Shakespeare and Chaucer mention ginger.

In the 1800s, a group of 25,000 physicians, collectively known as the Eclectics, popularized the medicinal uses of ginger in the United States. The *Materia Medica Therapeutics and Pharmacognosy* by Finley Ellingwood, M.D., included the many ways in which the Eclectics reported ginger to be of use in their medical practices.

Modern science has investigated the biochemical basis for ginger's illustrious history. It has broken this herb down to its most basic components and has discovered each component's effects, both separately and in combination with each other. The more you discover about ginger, the more you will see the benefits of this time-tested natural remedy.

Ginger Facts

Ginger was first harvested in Southeast Asia. Its scientific name, *Zingiber officinale,* was given by the famous Swedish botanist Linnaeus. It is a member of the *Zingiberacae* family, which also includes the healing herbs turmeric and cardamom (both found in curry, an Indian spice mixture). Through several linguistic twists and turns, the name "ginger" was derived from a Sanskrit word—*sringa-vera*—which describes its horn-like shape.

A graceful perennial, ginger can grow up to four feet in height. Its dark green leaves can extend to a foot in length and about three quarters of an inch wide. Many of the plants bud with sweet-smelling purple and yellow blossoms.

Although the edible part of ginger is often referred to as its root, botanists call it a *rhizome.* Rhizomes differ from roots in that they are able to bud and grow if split and planted. Carrots and potatoes are other examples of rhizomes. In this book, the terms "ginger" and "ginger root" are used interchangeably. Different varieties of ginger may be slightly different in shape and color, and they may vary widely in the composition of their medicinal components.

More than one hundred subspecies of ginger are grown throughout southern Asia, China, Jamaica, India, and other countries where the weather is warm and moist. Ginger, which requires healthy, rich soil, draws a great many nutrients into its rhizome as it grows. Most commercially available ginger is cultivated. It must be allowed to grow for at least six months to be useful, because it takes that long for the oils, which are believed to contain most of its medicinal components, to fully develop. Optimally, ginger should be allowed to grow and mature for nine months. At this point, it is bursting with over four hundred biochemicals, many of which are valuable healing agents.

Ginger As Medicine

Confucius wrote about ginger's benefits for aiding digestion, and two Chinese medical texts dating from 500 AD mention its medicinal uses. Western herbalists have made ginger a part of their natural pharmacies since the 1800s. The Hindu name for ginger is *vishwabhesaj,* which means "universal medicine." Today, it continues to be an important ingredient in many Asian and Ayurvedic herbal formulations.

In our modern medical age of laboratory-produced, chemical drugs, doctors and patients alike typically want more than a long history of or anecdotal evidence for natural remedies. They want clinical studies—scientific proof—that a remedy works.

Fortunately, a growing number of researchers are taking notice of ginger and are performing studies on this remarkable herb. Scientific knowledge and proof of ginger's therapeutic value is available now.

The whitish, fibrous flesh of the ginger rhizome has been analyzed exhaustively. It is made up of 12 to 50 percent carbohydrate (more mature plants contain more carbohydrate), 6 to 8 percent fat, 9 percent protein, and 2.5 percent fiber. Enzymes—most notably a protein-digesting enzyme called *zingibain*—make up between 2 and 3 percent of this edible portion of ginger. Zingibain can break down protein at an astonishing rate. One gram of zingibain can tenderize up to twenty pounds of meat. When eaten with meat, the zingibain in fresh ginger joins forces with the enzymes secreted in the stomach and small intestines, making digestion more thorough. It's no wonder that the cuisines of Asia and India include ginger in so many of their traditional meat dishes.

Ginger is rich in vitamins, minerals, and other *phytonutrients*—chemicals found in plants that support health. It is abundant in B vitamins (including niacin and thiamine), beta carotene, and vitamin C. Minerals found in ginger include calcium, chromium, germanium, iron, magnesium, phosphorus, selenium, and zinc. The amino acids arginine, cysteine, glycine, leucine, lysine, and tyrosine; and the health-supporting phytochemicals beta-sitosterol, capsaicin, curcumin, lecithin, limonene, and quercetin also are contained in ginger.

Volatile oils, also called *essential oils,* give ginger its taste and aroma. These oils, which vary between the different ginger subspecies and the soil in which they are grown, make up 1 to 3 percent of the average root. Possibly the most important health-supporting component of the ginger root is the sticky oil known as *oleoresin.* Oleoresins are where the magic of the ginger root lies. They contain hundreds of compounds that have a vast array of effects on the molecular machinery of the body. It's as though nature created this herb, according to precise specifications, to help maintain good health.

Ginger oleoresin's full spectrum of ingredients is lengthy, but its most fundamental constituents are the *gingerols.* Gingerols, of which there are more than twenty different types, make up approximately 33 percent of fresh ginger oleoresin. They are proving to be the most therapeutically valuable of ginger's chemical building blocks. You'll learn more about the beneficial effects of gingerols as you read on.

As scientists discover more about ginger's active ingredients, this knowledge is being used to create formulas for treating various health conditions. A number of researchers have been fascinated by ginger's positive effects on joint health. After meticulously testing the effects of each of ginger's active ingredients on joint health, one biochemist in particular, Dr. Morton Weidner, formulated an extract that is proving to be even more effective on arthritis and other inflammatory joint diseases than ginger root alone.

(Detailed information on the work of Dr. Weidner and other researchers is presented in Chapter 5.)

Scientists usually start with plant extracts and then attempt to isolate the active ingredients that have some therapeutic effect on the body. What these so-called "active" ingredients usually lack are the plant's *synergistic ingredients*—the other plant substances that help the active ingredients perform their functions. *Nutraceuticals* are natural therapeutic products that contain substances that exist in nature, but in order for them to be classified as prescription drugs, their active ingredients must be isolated in a lab. Once they have been chemically altered, they are unlike anything found in nature. This is the major difference between prescription arthritis drugs and nutraceuticals: nutraceuticals like ginger extract include synergistic ingredients necessary to optimize the health-promoting effects of the active ingredient, while prescription drugs are isolated compounds.

As previously discussed, the active ingredients of prescription drugs are often derived from plants. In order to create a "patentable" pharmaceutical, the manufacturer must somehow alter the molecules so that they are no longer completely natural. Most natural substances are not patentable, so they can't be priced competitively. Pharmaceutical companies end up changing the molecules into something the body doesn't recognize and something that isn't well-matched to the body's natural systems. This is one reason for the very high frequency of side effects seen with prescription drugs.

A Word About Extracts

Ginger extract typically is more expensive than powdered ginger or whole fresh ginger root. This is because it is standardized to the potency necessary for the desired effect. Standardized extracts are documented to contain a certain amount of the plant's active ingredients, so you know exactly what you're getting when you take them.

As mentioned earlier, ginger roots vary widely from species to species in their active ingredients. Processing further alters these ingredients. When you purchase a ginger powder or fresh root, or even a nonstandardized extract to ease the pain of arthritis, there's no guarantee that the product will produce the beneficial effects of a pure standardized extract. Finally, there is a reliable, well-researched, standardized ginger extract for treating inflammatory joint diseases.

Summing It Up

As you have learned through this chapter, ginger has a rich and ancient history. Its use as a medicine goes back to 200 BC. Within its fibrous, pungent rhizome lies an amazing array of medicinal constituents. The marriage of this ancient medicine with modern pharmaceutical science has given rise to a ginger extract designed specifically to treat inflammatory joint conditions such as arthritis. In the next chapter, we'll be taking a closer look at this often debilitating condition.

5.

Nature's Anti-Inflammatory

✳

Today, ginger is a component of over fifty different herbal remedies throughout the world. It has been used for centuries to relieve joint pain, headaches, sore throats, menstrual cramps, and toothaches.

The work of Danish researcher Dr. K. C. Srivastava in the 1980s provided sound scientific basis for ginger's role in easing the pain and inflammation of arthritis. His work has served as a springboard for many scientists, including biochemist Dr. Morton Weidner (introduced in Chapter 4), in isolating the ginger components that help relieve arthritis symptoms.

In one study involving laboratory rats with severely arthritic paws, Dr. Srivastava found that daily doses of ginger oil and eugenol—a constituent of ginger—significantly reduced the arthritis within thirty days. In a test-tube study, he found that the ginger extract reduced *lipoxygenase* formation. (As explained in

Chapter 2, lipoxygenase is the enzyme that creates "good" and "bad" leukotrienes and the COX-2 enzyme.) Another study involved fifty-six patients—twenty-eight with rheumatoid arthritis, eighteen with osteoarthritis, and ten with general muscle pain. After taking powdered ginger for a minimum of three months, all the patients experienced notable relief from their symptoms.

Dr. Weidner and Ginger Extract

Dr. Morton Weidner became interested in ginger as an arthritis remedy while working as a biochemist at the University of Copenhagen in Denmark. He realized how many people worldwide suffer from this disease, and he also knew the damaging side effects caused by the drugs normally prescribed for treating this condition. He saw the need for a natural product that could help control inflammation without negative side effects and committed himself to finding this remedy.

Starting his search in the medical library, he pored over scientific journals to discover which plants had been researched for their joint-healing potential. His next step was to travel the world collecting samples of these plants for in-depth analysis in his laboratory. He visited Africa, India, America, China, and Europe, tramping through jungles and climbing mountains to find his specimens. Back in Copenhagen, he analyzed the samples carefully to learn which ones had the most beneficial effects on arthritic joints. A species of ginger found in China showed the most promise.

Dr. Weidner spent six years and 4 million dollars researching and developing an extract from this ginger species. The result was a potent extract, composed of the phytochemicals in ginger that work synergistically to reverse the inflammatory process of arthritis. Dr. Weidner's method for extracting these chemicals from the ginger root is so unique, it has been patented. He also has developed the technology necessary for ensuring that the active ingredients are easily absorbed by the body in the digestive tract.

Dr. Weidner's extract is patented not because the ginger components have been altered to create synthetic versions, but because of the extraction and delivery processes that go into the making of each capsule. These processes ensure uniform amounts of active ingredients, and greatly enhance their absorption in the gastrointestinal tract.

Dr. Weidner's ginger extract may be purchased from Freelife: 800-359-3620; fax 203-882-7255; website www.FREELIFE.com.

Science and Nature Meet

Finally, a ginger formulation made from the parts of the ginger rhizome known to have the most potent anti-inflammatory effects is available. It has helped countless arthritis sufferers get off the prescription drug treadmill. The two species of ginger—*Zingiber officinale* and *Alpinia galanga*—used in this extract inhibit COX-2 enzymes and strongly inhibit 5-lipoxygenase. What's more, unlike NSAIDs, the extract works without causing any gastrointestinal side effects.

While NSAIDs, as seen in the last chapter, are designed to inhibit the action of COX enzymes, they don't have any significant effect on lipoxygenase. Over the last few years, a flurry of research has focused on the possible role of leukotrienes in inflammatory diseases. As previously mentioned, the "bad" versions of this eicosanoid can cause blood to thicken and free radicals to form. They also encourage an overabundance of immune cells and fluid in tender areas, causing inflammation.

As you saw in Chapter 2, the leukotriene eicosanoids exist in more than one form, just as cyclooxygenase enzymes do. Some are powerful stimulators of inflammation throughout the body, playing a significant role in the development of rheumatoid arthritis and inflammatory bowel disease. Other leukotrienes are linked to the chronic constriction and inflammation of airways that are the hallmarks of asthma. Drugs that inhibit leukotrienes are prescribed to asthma patients in an attempt to control their symptoms, and, in about half of these cases, it works well. Of course, as with any prescription drug, there is always the risk of side effects, including headache, dizziness, abdominal pain, general weakness, and vomiting, as well as dangerous interactions with other drugs.

During his research, Dr. Weidner discovered that while cyclooxygenase did play a role in short-term joint discomfort, long-term joint discomfort was caused by leukotrienes. He then exhaustively analyzed ginger's constituents, one at a time, to discover which of them would inhibit COX enzymes and which would inhibit 5-lipoxygenase, the enzyme that creates strongly pro-inflammatory leukotrienes.

When he had finished his analyses, Dr. Weidner looked at the effectiveness of his finished product in laboratory studies. First, he tested the effects of the ginger extract on the rate of prostaglandin formation from arachidonic acid—the raw material from which "bad" prostaglandins are made. He found that the extract inhibited the rate at which these prostaglandins were created from arachidonic acid by about 20 percent.

Dr. Weidner then repeated the experiment, this time focusing on the extract's effects on leukotriene synthesis from arachidonic acid. The ginger extract had an amazing inhibitory effect on 5-lipoxygenase, inhibiting "bad" leukotriene production by nearly 100 percent! It is the first product to slow the formation of *both* prostaglandins and leukotrienes.

Inflammation and Free Radicals

Free radicals, as discussed in detail in Chapter 2, accelerate the inflammatory process. Immune cells gathering at the site of inflammation stimulate the formation of inflammatory eicosanoids, which, in turn, cause more free radicals to form. Free radicals are destructive to joint tissues and to *hyaluronic acid*—the slippery joint-protective fluid that prevents damaging friction in the joints. Antioxidant substances from the ginger rhizome interrupt this cycle, helping to prevent free-radical formation from spinning out of control.

Dr. Weidner investigated the effects of ginger extract on the sudden increase in the formation of free radicals that occurs with inflammation. This "oxidative burst" is a major culprit in the permanent joint damage that occurs with arthritis. He found that at the recommended dose, ginger extract reduced the oxidative burst by about 25 percent.

Tumor necrosis factor-alpha (TNF-α) and interleukin1-beta (IL1-β)—a "bad" interleukin—are powerful inducers of inflammation. They also stimulate certain chemicals that break down collagen (the basic building block of cartilage) and generate pain. When a joint with arthritis is regularly stressed, it pumps out copious amounts of TNF-α. This doesn't happen in response to mechanical stress in a joint that does not have arthritis. In osteoarthritis patients, higher than normal levels of TNF-α are found in the joint fluid and membranes. Ginger extract was found to stifle the inflammatory actions of "bad" interleukins and TNF-α.

When joints become inflamed and TNF-α and IL1-β are released, *chondrocytes* (cartilage-making cells) begin to make a particularly dangerous type of free radical called *nitric oxide*. Nitric oxide, in turn, shuts down collagen synthesis, causing cartilage to die off. In test-tube studies, ginger extract dampened the free radical fire of nitric oxide.

Ginger extract also stimulates the body's production of IL-4 and IL-10—"good" interleukins that encourage the rebuilding of tissues destroyed by inflammation.

The Studies

To date, there have been a number of pilot studies documenting the effectiveness of ginger extract for the relief of arthritis pain and inflammation.

In a three-month study, Danish scientist Dr. M. Norgard researched the effects of ginger extract on twenty-eight subjects who had suffered with chronic joint pain from seven to thirty-five years. By the end of the study, twenty-five displayed significant improvement. And none reported any side effects.

Another Danish scientist, Dr. Henning Bliddal, led a study at the Copenhagen Municipal Hospital. Fifty-six subjects with arthritis participated. Half of the participants were given the ginger extract, and the other half were given a placebo (sugar pill). Halfway through the study, the groups were switched, so that each group had a chance to take the ginger extract. (The subjects did not know what they were taking at any point during the study.) The results showed no change in the range of motion of the affected joints, but subjects experienced significant pain relief while taking the ginger extract compared to those using the placebo. No side effects were observed.

In Singapore, Dr. Leong Keng Hong compared the effects of the ginger extract with a placebo in sixty-two arthritis sufferers. Those using the ginger extract found their symptoms had improved in only three weeks' time. There were no reports of any adverse effects.

A ten-week study conducted in the United States analyzed the effects of ginger extract on 140 patients with arthritic knees. Half of the subjects were given ginger extract, while the other half were given a placebo. Those taking the ginger extract displayed significant improvement in knee pain compared to those taking the placebo. Again, there were no side effects.

Ginger's Effects on Other Conditions

Ginger root has been used medicinally for centuries. Not only is it effective in controlling joint pain and inflammation, it is both a preventive and a remedy for other types of pain, including migraine headaches and menstrual cramps. *Phytochemicals*—substances in plants that have various health-promoting properties—that are found in the ginger rhizome may even prove important in the fight against cancer and heart disease. Ginger is also enormously beneficial to the digestive tract—so much so that Chapter 6 is devoted entirely to this subject.

Inflammation, Heart Disease, and Cancer

According to long-term studies involving the effects of NSAIDs on subjects with joint inflammation, the subjects also experienced very few incidents of cancer and heart disease. This caused researchers to investigate possible connections between runaway inflammation and the two most dangerous diseases in Western countries—heart disease and cancer.

Constricted blood vessels are a major factor in heart attacks, strokes, and chronic high blood pressure. In addition to being caused by clogged blood vessels that feed the heart, heart attacks are caused by the constriction of partially clogged blood vessels. This is especially true for women.

In addition to constricted blood vessels, heart attacks and strokes also are linked to thickened blood, which typically results in dangerous blood clots. This, in turn, increases the likelihood of clogged blood vessels. Eicosanoid imbalace allows "bad" eicosanoids to cause blood components to stick together, resulting in clots. This means a greater risk of heart disease and stroke. And although NSAIDs have been effective in helping maintain the proper blood fluidity, their negative side effects on the gastrointestinal tract cannot be denied. This is another reason that treatment with ginger extract is so attractive. It has the same positive effects of NSAIDs without the harmful side effects.

Some constituents of the ginger root also are known to have cancer-preventive effects. This may be due partly to its antioxidant properties and partly to its balancing effects on eicosanoids. Since the 1970s, scientists have toyed with the idea of a link between cancer and inflammation. Deaths from colon cancer were decreased by half in large study groups in which the subjects took aspirin daily to prevent heart attacks. In another study of 2,045 women, frequent use of NSAIDs decreased breast cancer risk. And the more often NSAIDs were used, the lower the risk became. Inhibiting "bad" eicosanoids appears to have an effect against the development of cancer. Once again, because ginger extract has the anti-inflammatory efficacy of NSAIDs—without the side effects—it is clearly a better choice.

Rising cancer rates also are believed to be linked to our ever-increasing exposure to carcinogenic chemicals in the environment. Some of these chemicals become carcinogenic only when they react with certain enzymes in the gastrointestinal tract. Many of these enzymes are the same ones responsible for the formation of "bad" eicosanoids. When we inhibit these enzymes, we inhibit the formation of certain dangerous carcinogens.

Chronic Pain

Traditionally, ginger has been used for coping with and controlling chronic pain. It is believed to work by inhibiting COX-2 enzymes and any other substance that carries the chemical message of pain through the nervous system. Studies on laboratory animals have supported the use of ginger for the relief of pain from headaches, body aches, and even menstrual cramps.

Certain ginger phytochemicals inhibit the release of *substance P,* a nervous system chemical that causes us to feel pain. They also inhibit the release of an enzyme called *thromboxane synthetase,* which is necessary for the manufacturing of a type of thromboxane that increases sensations of pain. When thromboxane synthetase is inhibited, the body releases another kind of hormone called *endorphins.* Endorphins are natural pain relievers. Pain relief from the use of ginger extract is, therefore, likely due to a combination of the inhibition of COX-2 enzymes, the inhibition of thromboxane synthetase, and the stimulation of endorphins.

Migraine Headache

Migraine headaches affect 6 percent of American men and 18 percent of American women. According to figures from the Centers for Disease Control, the prevalence of migraine headaches has risen more than 60 percent since 1981.

Over half of all migraine sufferers have a family history of the condition, and they tend to experience these blindingly painful headaches between the ages of twenty and thirty-five. Intense nausea, vomiting, and dizziness often accompany migraines. In some cases, certain warning signs precede the onset of an attack, including tingling or numbness in the body, disorientation, or extreme fatigue. Some people see sparks of light or auras around people just before a migraine begins. The pain of these headaches can be intense and debilitating.

Unfortunately, causes of migraines and how to cure them are still unknown. Some research points to an overreactive system of blood vessels in the brain. Arteries are not just hollow tubes through which blood flows; they are well-muscled walls that narrow and expand in response to stimulation from the nervous and hormonal systems. During a migraine, the blood vessels just inside the skull constrict strongly, reducing blood flow to a trickle. They then suddenly expand, causing the nerves along the carotid artery to compress, resulting in this type of intense headache. It makes sense that eicosanoid imbalances could cause these blood vessel changes. Changes in the electrical activity of the brain also are believed to cause blood vessel constriction. Inflammation of blood vessels in the brain also has been noted in migraine sufferers. The release of certain neurotransmitters from one of the cranial nerves causes inflammation, resulting in headache pain. Most likely, migraine headaches are caused by a combination of these and, possibly, other factors.

In Ayurvedic medicine, ginger has a long history of neurological benefits. It helps maintain proper eicosanoid balance, prevent blood from clotting, and block the effects of substance P. In addition, ginger eases two of the characteristic symptoms of migraine headaches—nausea and vomiting.

Menstrual Pain

A number of factors are implicated in the painful, sometimes debilitating cramps associated with menstruation. Typically, many women turn to NSAIDs or synthetic estrogens for relief. Researcher Dr. Joshua Backon observed that the prescription drug Clonidine has been shown to be effective in relieving menstrual cramps. This drug inhibits thromboxane synthetase and stimulates the release of the body's natural pain-killing endorphins. As you have seen earlier, ginger has the same inhibiting effects as Clonidine on thromboxane synthetase. The difference is that ginger is a natural remedy and causes no side effects.

Summing It Up

Ginger has huge untapped potential as a natural remedy for inflammatory conditions. The development of an effective ginger extract is popularizing its efficacy in the treatment of these conditions. The extract's many active components have a balancing, equalizing effect on the body, bringing pro- and anti-inflammatory hormones into proper balance. The antioxidants that occur naturally in the ginger rhizome help break the cycle of free-radical formation that can be so damaging in chronic inflammation. And what makes ginger extract so much more attractive than NSAIDs is that it can relieve the pain and inflammation of arthritic joints without the common side effects that accompany drugs.

In addition to its effectiveness in combating the pain and discomfort of inflammatory conditions, ginger also is helpful in promoting a healthy digestive tract. And among other things, a healthy digestive system has a direct impact on joint health. The next chapter presents this aspect of ginger's positive influence on health.

6

Ginger for a Healthy Digestive System

✳

Throughout this book, you've seen how ginger has been used over the centuries for a wide variety of conditions. In this chapter, you'll discover its effectiveness on the digestive system. You'll also see how prescription and over-the-counter medications commonly used for treating arthritis can cause a number of gastrointestinal problems, such as ulcers. Finally, you'll learn the connection between a healthy digestive system and healthy joints.

A healthy digestive tract, which includes the esophagus, stomach, small intestine, and colon (also referred to as the large intestine) is an integral part of a healthy body. The liver, gallbladder, and pancreas also play important roles in the digestive process. In simple terms, this system is designed to absorb important nutrients found in foods and eliminate any waste. When this system does not work efficiently, toxins build up and organs don't function as they should. To illustrate the importance of a healthy digestive system, let's compare it to the plumbing system that brings water to and from your home. If the plumbing is working properly, sufficient water enters the system at just the right temperature and pressure, while the waste water drains efficiently from kitchen sinks, toilets, and washing machines. If, however, even a small section of this system isn't working, your home can become a very unpleasant place to live. Everything from doing the laundry to brushing teeth to taking a shower can become a challenge.

Ginger's most common, traditional medicinal uses are for soothing upset stomachs and promoting proper digestion. Who hasn't been advised to sip a glass of ginger ale to help settle a queasy stomach? In addition to relieving nausea and vomiting, whether caused by pregnancy, surgery, motion sickness, or reactions to drug treatments such as chemotherapy, ginger also is a proven remedy for stomach ulcers and indigestion. Furthermore, it upholds the well-being of the small intestine and colon. Before detailing ginger's positive impact on a healthy digestive system, which also has a connection to healthy joints, let's begin with a brief overview of the digestive process.

The Working of the Digestive System

The digestive process begins in the mouth. When we chew food, it mixes with saliva, which contains enzymes that begin to break down carbohydrates. Through wavy muscular contractions known as *peristalsis,* the food makes its way from the mouth to the stomach via the esophagus. A sphincter muscle located at the bottom of the esophagus regulates the passage of food into the stomach.

The stomach is a muscular-walled organ lined with *parietal cells,* which are responsible for releasing *hydrochloric acid* (HCl). Hydrochloric acid kills bacteria and begins breaking down food. Other stomach cells secrete *pepsin,* a protein-digesting enzyme. The stomach walls rhythmically contract, thoroughly mixing HCl and pepsin with the food you've just enjoyed.

Pepsin and HCl work cooperatively in the digestive process. The right amount of HCl is needed to activate pepsin. Maintaining the proper acid-alkaline level (more commonly known as the pH level) within the stomach is extremely important. When the proper level is reached, signals are sent to eicosanoid-secreting cells in the stomach.

As mentioned in an earlier chapter, certain eicosanoids secrete mucus to protect the stomach lining. Hydrochloric acid also helps liberate B vitamins and minerals, such as potassium and magnesium, so they can be absorbed through the walls of the small intestine.

Pepsin is the only digestive enzyme secreted in the stomach. Other enzymes, including *protease* for digesting proteins, *amylase* for digesting starches, *lipase* for digesting fat, *lactase* for digesting lactose from dairy products, and *cellulase* for digesting cellulose from plant fiber, are manufactured in the small intestine. Pepsin does more than simply break down the protein components of the foods we eat. The breakdown products of protein, called *peptides,* stimulate specific hormones and nerve responses in the stomach, encouraging enhanced motility of the partially digested food. Good motility means short transit time through the digestive process, which, generally, is a good thing.

To sum it up, our bodies need the right amount of stomach acid (HC1) to trigger adequate secretion of pepsin and eicosanoids. This keeps the stomach lining healthy and encourages proper transit time of the digested food. Slow transit time usually indicates a sluggish digestive system that is overworked. It commonly results in bloating, constipation, and feeling fatigued. Heartburn, also called *gastroesophageal reflux,* is another common sign of slow transit time. It occurs when the sphincter muscle at the base of the esophagus allows partly digested food from the stomach to back up into the esophagus. A healthy stomach has a thick mucus lining to protect it from this acidic mixture, but the esophagus doesn't have such protection. The result is a burning sensation. Large, fatty meals, which tend to sit in the stomach for relatively long periods of time, are more likely to cause heartburn. They also encourage slow transit time. Another problem with slow transit time is that it allows toxins that are intended for elimination to sit too long in the digestive tract. These toxins can be absorbed into the body through the walls of the small intestine or colon, or they may do damage to the cells that line these organs.

On the other hand, very fast transit time during digestion isn't desirable either because the body isn't able to absorb the nutrients from food properly. Food that rushes through the digestive tract usually results in diarrhea. In most cases, however, diarrhea is the way in which the body tries to expel something that may cause illness. Unless it is chronic or very severe, diarrhea is best left alone to run its course.

Another sphincter muscle acts as a gatekeeper between the stomach and the small intestine. Once the contents of the stomach reach a certain pH level, the sphincter muscle opens, allowing small squirts of the stomach's contents into the duodenum—the first part of the small intestine. This area is where the pancreas is located. In addition to its job of manufacturing insulin, the pancreas releases enzymes into the small intestine to continue the digestive process.

Under a microscope, the lining of the twenty-two-foot-long small intestine looks like a plush carpet. Throughout its twists and turns are minuscule protrusions called villi. Each of the villi contains a network of capillaries through which nutrients are absorbed. The nutrients are then carried into the bloodstream and used by the body.

Bile, which is made in the liver and stored in the gallbladder, is released into the small intestines to further aid in the digestive process. Acting as an emulsifier, bile breaks down fats. Proper fat digestion means faster transit time and better absorption of nutrients. It also means less chance of indigestion from incompletely digested fats.

Next, the waste matter passes into the colon. This organ is responsible for reabsorbing water and minerals back into the body, then eliminating the remaining waste. The colon also houses colonies of "friendly" bacteria, also called *probiotics*. Several strains of probiotics perform a wide variety of important duties. Some cultures manufacture B vitamins, which are then absorbed into the body through the colon wall. Other forms are responsible for keeping infectious, "bad" bacteria and harmful yeasts at bay. Probiotics also help prevent constipation and neutralize toxins that can cause illness, including colon cancer. If food is not completely digested when it reaches the colon, "friendly" bacteria help to finish the job, creating intestinal gas and bloating in the process. Any remaining waste material is eliminated from the body.

Ginger's Effects on the Digestive System

Certain properties of ginger encourage proper digestion, so it has long been a useful remedy in easing and preventing disorders of the gastrointestinal tract. Most commonly, ginger is used to ease nausea and vomiting, but it also is effective in treating stomach ulcers and other digestive system conditions.

An Aid for Ulcers

For many years, excess stomach acid was believed to be the only cause of stomach and duodenal ulcers. It is true that studies have shown that those with duodenal ulcers have twice as many acid-producing cells as do those without this type of ulcer. However, those with gastric ulcers, which are located in the stomach, actually have normal or lower than normal stomach acid secretions. What scientists have discovered is that the use of NSAIDs, coffee, and tobacco are likely contributors to the formation of gastric ulcers. An estimated one-third of the cases of bleeding ulcers are specifically attributed to continuous NSAID use.

Recently, scientists at the University of Virginia discovered another cause of ulcers—a spiral-shaped bacteria called *Helicobacter pylori* (*H. pylori*). Found to be a major factor in many cases of ulcer, *H. pylori* attacks and wears away the mucus that protects the stomach and duodenal walls from digestive acids. Since antibiotics kill *H. pylori,* they are generally part of the drug treatment for ulcers. Ginger extract is helpful in combating *H. pylori* in two ways. First, ginger has antibiotic properties itself, and second, it enhances the effectiveness of prescription antibiotics.

For preventing excess stomach acid in many ulcer patients, physicians commonly recommend antacids or histamine (H2) blockers. Antacids neutralize existing stomach acid, and H2 blockers, such as cimetidine (Tagamet) and ranitidine (Zantac) decrease the production of stomach acid. These drugs are among the top-selling ulcer drugs in the United States. Physicians also prescribe H2 blockers for the treatment of heartburn, and they are available over the counter. Both antacids and H2 blockers are often prescribed to those who are at risk for developing NSAID-related ulcers.

Using H2 blockers and antacids may help ease the discomfort of ulcers and heartburn, but not without a price. As you have seen, a certain amount of stomach acid is important for proper digestion. Decreasing this level disrupts the process. Acid-reducing drugs can result in incomplete food breakdown, compromised nutrient absorption, and decreased motility in moving food along the gastrointestinal tract. Worse, in many cases, these drugs mask the symptoms of ulcers, allowing them to progress. Remember what happened to our friend Hugh in Chapter 3?

Ginger extract is a safe, effective alternative to these drugs. Its components actually help to balance stomach acidity and pepsin secretion, rather than shutting them down like ulcer drugs. And most important, ginger causes no harmful side effects.

Other Positive Effects

In addition to its important role in preventing ulcers and easing stomach upset, ginger extract is helpful in the proper absorption of nutrients in the small intestine. Ginger's constituents naturally are absorbed very rapidly through this intestinal lining. When it is taken along with food, the extract "carries" the food's nutrients with it as it is absorbed through the small intestine. In the same way, when ginger is taken with medicine, it "carries" the medicine's healing properties with it through the intestinal wall. This is one of the reasons ginger is added to so many different herbal remedies—it increases the absorption and potency of the other ingredients.

Ginger also helps enhance the body's production of bile, which further aids proper digestion. It also promotes proper transit time of digested matter. In the colon, ginger has soothing properties that help ease intestinal spasms that cause cramping. Finally, its antibacterial components support probiotic levels, encouraging their growth in the intestinal tract.

The Link Between Your Gut and Your Joints

So you have seen that ginger has a number of positive effects on the gastrointestinal system. What does this have to do with healthy joints? The answer lies primarily in ginger's effect on the small intestine.

The lining of the small intestine is designed to be extremely selective. It absorbs only what the body needs and eliminates what it doesn't. At least, this is what occurs in a healthy small intestine. Prescription drugs (particularly NSAIDs), food allergies, and poor diets that rely heavily on processed foods are the biggest culprits in eroding the intestinal lining. Eventually, this causes the formation of tiny leaks—a condition known as leaky gut syndrome. As seen in Chapter 1, this condition allows partially digested bits of food and chemical toxins to permeate the intestinal lining, where they enter the bloodstream. The immune system then springs into action and attacks these "foreign" invaders. However, when the immune system has to fight these invaders constantly, it gets tired and eventually is compromised. Leaky gut is associated with a number of autoimmune diseases, such as irritable bowel syndrome, chronic allergies, asthma, chronic fatigue, and arthritis.

Dozens of studies have indicated that both rheumatoid arthritis and osteoarthritis are attributable, at least in part, to food allergies. The Western diet largely consists of foods such as corn, eggs, beef, nightshade vegetables (potatoes, tomatoes, peppers, eggplant), white flour, soy, and dairy products, and other foods that may be allergenic to certain individuals. When these foods are eaten too often, the small intestines begin to mount an immune response that can result in leaky gut syndrome. When this happens, and allergenic substances are able to permeate the "leaks" in the intestinal lining, they may become lodged in the joint tissues. Then the immune system causes an inflammatory response in the joint. This can be the cause of arthritis or it can exacerbate an already existing arthritic condition.

To discover whether your arthritis has been caused or aggravated by food allergies, an elimination diet is suggested. Begin this simple diet by writing a list of the foods you eat every day. Include the foods you crave on a regular basis and feel you cannot live without. These are the foods to which you are probably sensitive. *Nightshade vegetables,* such as tomatoes, potatoes, peppers, and eggplants, often are implicated in arthritis caused by food allergy.

The next step is to eliminate these foods completely from your diet for at least two weeks. Replace the foods you eliminate with fresh whole foods like vegetables (not including nightshade varieties), whole grains, and beans. If wheat is one of the foods to be eliminated, all other grains that contain gluten— oats, millet, barley, rye, spelt, and amaranth—must be eliminated as well. Keep a journal during this diet and keep track of your symptoms. It is likely that you will notice some improvement in the first few days.

Once you have gone through the elimination period, it's time to challenge your body by reintroducing the foods one at a time. Introduce only one food during a twenty-four-hour period, and then have *only* that food for a meal. For example, if you have eliminated wheat from your diet, do not choose to eat bread, because it contains many other ingredients besides wheat. Instead, have a bowl of cream of wheat or cooked wheat berries. Keep track of any symptoms you may experience after eating the food. If you notice that your joints start to ache or that you experience some other reaction, eliminate the food again for another four weeks, then try again. If, on the other hand, there is no reaction to the newly introduced food, you can feel confident in adding it back in your diet. Keep reintroducing each food from the list, one at a time, until you determine exactly which foods cause reactions.

Don't despair if you have to eliminate your favorite foods. Feeling better should make it worthwhile. After a time, you will probably be able to enjoy that food once in a while as an occasional treat. For more information on elimination diets, read *Optimal Wellness* by Ralph Golan, M.D. (New York: Ballantine Books, 1992).

Summing It Up

Commonly prescribed arthritis drugs may ease arthritis symptoms, but are commonly a major cause of digestive distress. The problem is that many patients believe they have no choice—that they must compromise their digestive health for joint health. The good news is that ginger extract offers a safe, effective alternative to drugs for arthritis sufferers. Always a natural medicine of choice for stomach problems, ginger—in a patented extract form—offers arthritis sufferers the best of both worlds. It helps heal joints while keeping the gastrointestinal system strong.

A Final Word

*

The ginger rhizome is one of nature's most abundant sources of healing plant chemicals. Over centuries of use and research, modern science is rediscovering what sages of old already knew—that ginger is an effective remedy for arthritis, aches and pains, migraine, menstrual cramps, and intestinal and stomach complaints.

With all the finesse modern pharmaceutical science has to offer, nutritional research has provided us with ginger extracts containing potent anti-inflammatory, eicosanoid-balancing ingredients. I predict ginger extract someday will be as well-known and as widely used as aspirin is today.

Ginger extract isn't a miracle cure. It is a sensible, effective alternative to NSAID drugs that tear up the gastrointestinal tract. It is a gentle pain reliever that helps people who have been in chronic pain to live active, fulfilling lives once again. There are no side effects to contend with, and even the creators of the fast-selling COX-2 inhibitor can't say this about their product.

It also looks as though balancing eicosanoids with ginger extract could prevent all kinds of disease processes from moving forward. Heart disease and cancer are two of the most feared diseases known to man, and scientists are now linking those diseases to out-of-balance eicosanoids. Most of the research you'll see about balancing these hormones will focus on the prescription NSAIDs, especially the COX-2 inhibitors. You can balance eicosanoids just as effectively—and far more safely—with ginger extract.

Glossary

✳

Adrenaline. A hormone, also called *epinephrine,* that is released by the adrenal glands in response to stress, exercise, or strong emotion. Chronic high levels can cause insulin levels to rise, resulting in eicosanoid imbalance.

Antioxidant. A naturally occurring substance produced in the body and in some plants that counteracts the harmful effects of free radicals. Examples include vitamins C and E, beta-carotene, and many constituents of ginger root.

Autoimmune disease. A condition in which the immune system attacks the body's own tissues, interfering with normal functioning. Examples include rheumatoid arthritis, ulcerative colitis, and lupus.

Arachidonic acid. A type of fatty acid from which "bad" eicosanoids are made.

Cartilage. The smooth protective tissue that cushions the ends of bones, reducing friction at the joints. Degeneration leads to osteoarthritis.

Chondrocytes. Cartilage-making cells.

Collagen. A fibrous protein that is the primary constituent of bone, cartilage, and connective tissue. It is the most abundant protein in the body.

Cortisol. A hormone secreted by the adrenal glands in response to stress, hunger, and exercise. Chronic high levels can adversely affect eicosanoid balance.

Cyclooxygenases. Enzymes that transform activated fatty acids (GLA and DHGLA) into prostaglandins.

Cytokines. Immune cells that stimulate the inflammatory response.

Delta 5-desaturase. An enzyme that transforms activated fatty acids into eicosapentaenoic and arachidonic acids. Proper nutrition decreases delta-5 activity. This, in turn, helps decrease the formation of "bad" eicosanoids from omega-6 fats, improving eicosanoid balance.

Delta 6-desaturase. An enzyme that transforms essential fats into activated fatty acids, GLA and DHGLA; this enzyme is suppressed by high cortisol and adrenaline levels caused by stress, which can disrupt eicosanoid balance.

Dihomo-gamma-linoleic acid (DHGLA). An activated fatty acid that is created when delta 6-desaturase acts on linoleic acids from omega-6 oils.

Duodenum. The first section of the small intestine that begins at the lower end of the stomach. It is about 25 centimeters long.

Eicosanoids. Short-lived hormones that act on cells. They consist of three groups—prostaglandins, leukotrienes, and thromboxanes—which are effective in preventing blood clots, inflammation, and high blood pressure. They are important for gastrointestinal health and the health of the immune system.

Eicosapentaenoic acid (EPA). The healthful fat that is created when delta 5- and delta 6-desaturase enzymes act on omega-3 oils. It is then transformed by cyclooxygenases and lipoxygenases to "good" prostaglandins and leukotrienes.

Endorphins. Hormone-like substances that are natural painkillers and mood enhancers. They are found primarily in the brain.

Essential fatty acids (EFAs). Fatty acids necessary for health that are obtained only through diet. Omega-3 and omega-6 are the two types.

Free radicals. An atom or group of atoms with at least one unpaired electron, making it highly unstable. Free radicals join readily with other substances and can cause damage at the cellular level. They are the result of normal metabolism, as well as the result of exposure to radiation, pollutants, and the inflammatory process. They are blocked by antioxidants.

Gamma-linoleic acid (GLA). Linoleic acids from omega-6 fats that have been acted upon by delta 6-desaturase enzyme.

Gastric. Having to do with the stomach.

Gingerols. The most potent constituents of ginger oleoresin.

Helicobacter pylori (H. pylori). Bacteria that grows in the mucus-secreting cells of the stomach lining. It is a common cause of gastritis.

Hydrochloric acid (HCl). The strong acid secreted by the stomach to aid in the digestion of food.

Hyaluronic acid. A natural joint-protective compound. It is destroyed by free radicals that are created during inflammation.

Inflammation. An immune response to infection or injury in which immune cells and fluid are brought to the affected area. It is characterized by swelling, heat, and redness. Inflammation can result in tissue damage if not controlled by proper eicosanoid balance.

Interleukins. Part of the immune system that helps regulate an immune response. They play a key role in regulating inflammation.

Leaky gut. A condition in which food sensitivities lead to inflammation in the small intestine, causing small holes to form. Partially digested food particles and toxins pass through these leaks and enter the bloodstream, eventually compromising the body's immune system. Leaky gut is associated with a number of autoimmune conditions such as asthma, chronic fatigue, and arthritis.

Leukotriene. A type of eicosanoid that helps regulate inflammation, immunity, mucus secretion, and muscle contraction.

Lipoxygenases. A group of enzymes responsible for the formation of "good" and "bad" leukotrienes.

Lymphocytes. Immune cells; important in regulating the inflammatory process.

Motility. The speed at which food moves through the digestive tract.

Natural killer cell. Type of immune cell that can kill certain cancer cells.

Nitric oxide. A chemical made in the body that relaxes muscles in blood vessel walls, allowing them to open.

Non-steroidal anti-inflammatory drugs (NSAIDs). Any of a class of over-the-counter or prescription drugs that are commonly used to relieve mild to moderate pain.

Oleoresin. The sticky part of the ginger rhizome that contains most of its active ingredients.

Omega-3 fats. Essential fats found in fish oils and certain vegetable oils, including canola and flaxseed. They are the raw material for "good" eicosanoids.

Omega-6 fats. Essential fats found in unsaturated oils, such as black currant, borage, evening primrose, grapeseed, sesame seed, and soybean; also present in raw nuts, seeds, and legumes. They are the raw material for both "good" and "bad" eicosanoids.

Osteoarthritis. The most common form of arthritis in which the cartilage that cushions joints begins to wear. It is believed to be caused primarily by wear and tear.

Oxidation. A chemical reaction in which oxygen reacts with another substance, often resulting in some type of spoilage. This process causes free radicals.

Pepsin. An enzyme secreted in the stomach that breaks down proteins during digestion. Most ulcer drugs decrease pepsin's action, adversely affecting digestion.

Peristalsis. Rhythmic muscular contractions of the gastrointestinal tract that move food along during the digestive process.

Platelets. Components of blood responsible for clotting.

Probiotics. Strains of "friendly" bacteria that colonize in the gastrointestinal tract. They manufacture B vitamins, aid in the digestive process, and neutralize toxins and carcinogens.

Prostacyclin. A "good" prostaglandin that maintains proper blood fluidity and dilates blood vessels. Celebrex, commonly prescribed for arthritis, suppresses its formation.

Prostaglandin. Type of eicosanoid that affects pain sensations, inflammation, body temperature, the constriction and expansion of blood vessels, blood clotting, and the health of the stomach lining. It also plays a key role in regulating body temperature, expanding and contracting blood vessels, and maintaining proper blood fluidity and healthy stomach lining.

Phytochemicals. Any one of a number of substances found in plants that have various health-promoting properties, including protection against certain types of cancer.

Rheumatoid arthritis. An autoimmune disorder in which the immune system mistakenly attacks the body's own tissues, causing chronic inflammation, pain, and joint swelling.

Rhizome. Root-like part of a plant that is able to bud and grow if split and replanted.

Serotonin. A neurotransmitter that is important for regulating a number of functions, including mood, relaxation, sleep, and concentration. Because of its interactions with platelets and substance P, it may play a role in causing migraine headaches.

Substance P. A chemical produced in the body that stimulates the sensation of pain.

Thromboxanes. Eicosanoids responsible for the regulation of blood clotting and pain responses.

Thromboxane synthetase. An enzyme needed to make thromboxanes. Increased levels suppress the formation of endorphins, while decreased levels encourage it.

Transit time. The amount of time necessary for the digestive process to take place, from start to finish.

Zingibain. Protein-digesting enzyme found in ginger root.

References

*

1. The Arthritis Epidemic

Brooks, P. M., S. R. Potter, and W. W. Buchanan. "NSAIDs and osteoarthritis—help or hindrance?" *Journal of Rheumatology,* 1982; 9:3–5.

Darlington, L. G., N. W. Ramsey, and J. R. Mansfield. "Placebo-controlled, blind study of dietary manipulation in rheumatoid arthritis." *Lancet,* 1986; i:236–38.

Newman, N. M., and R. S. M. Ling. "Acetabular bond destruction related to non-steroidal anti-inflammatory drugs." *Lancet,* 1985; ii:11–13.

Petersdorf, R., et al. *Harrison's Principles of Internal Medicine.* New York: McGraw-Hill, 1983.

Pizzorno, J. E., and M. Murray. *A Textbook of Natural Medicine.* Seattle, WA: John Bastyr College Publications, 1985.

Segal, A.W., et al. "Preliminary evidence for gut involvement in the pathogenesis of rheumatoid arthritis." *British Journal of Rheumatology,* 1986; 25:162–66.

Smith, M. D., R. A. Gibson, and P. M. Brooks. "Abnormal bowel permeability in ankylosing spondylitis and rheumatoid arthritis." *Journal of Rheumatology,* 1985; 12:299–305.

Zaphiropoulos, G. C. "Rheumatoid arthritis and the gut." *British Journal of Rheumatology,* 1986; 25:138–40.

2. Inflammation and Eicosanoids

Alexander, J. W. "Immunonutrition: the role of omega-3 fatty acids." *Nutrition,* July/August 1998; 14(7–8):627–33.

Belch, J. F., et al. "Effects of altering dietary essential fatty acids on requirements for nonsteroidal anti-inflammatory drugs in patients with rheumatoid arthritis: a double blind placebo controlled study." *Annals of Rheumatic Diseases,* 1988; 47:96–104.

Berry, E. M., and J. Hirsch. "Does dietary linolenic acid influence blood pressure?" *American Journal of Clinical Nutrition,* 1986; 44:336–40.

Blond, J. P., and P. Lemarchel. "A study on the effect of alpha linolenic acid on the desaturation of dihomo-gamma-linolenic acids using rat liver homogenates." *Reproductive Nutrition Development,* 1984; 24:1–10.

Borkman, M., et al. "The relationship between insulin sensitivity and the fatty acid composition of skeletal muscle phospholipids." *New England Journal of Medicine,* 1993; 328:238–44.

Brenner, R. R. "Nutritional and hormonal factors influencing desaturation of essential fatty acids." *Progressive Lipid Research,* 1982; 20:41–48.

Coulston, A. M., G. C. Liu, and G. M. Reaven. "Plasma, glucose, insulin and lipid responses to high-carbohydrate, low-fat diets in normal humans." *Metabolism,* 1983; 32:52–56.

Cunnane, S. C., et al. "Alpha-linolenic acid in humans: direct functional role or dietary precursor?" *Nutrition,* 1991; 7:437–39.

Hamilton, L. C., et al. "Synergy between cyclo-oxygenase-2 induction and arachidonic acid supply in vivo: consequences for nonsteroidal anti-inflammatory drug efficacy." *FASEB Journal,* February 1999; 13(2):245–51.

Hill, E. G., et al. "Perturbation of the metabolism of essential fatty acids by dietary partially hydrogenated vegetable oil." *Proceedings of the National Academy of Sciences, USA,* 1982; 79:953–57.

Kelley, D. S. "Alpha-linolenic acid and immune response." *Nutrition,* 1992; 8:215–17.

Kremer, J., et al. "Effects of manipulation of dietary fatty acids on clinical manifestation of rheumatoid arthritis." *Lancet,* 1985; i:184–87.

Maslinka, D., and M. Gajewski. "Some aspects of the inflammatory process." *Folia Neuropathologica,* 1998; 36(4):199–204.

Murray, Michael T. *Encyclopedia of Nutritional Supplements.* Rocklin, CA: Prima Publishing, 1996.

Nettleton, J. A. "Omega-3 fatty acids: comparison of plant and seafood sources in human nutrition." *Journal of the American Dietary Association,* 1991; 91:331–37.

Pelikanova, T., et al. "Insulin secretion and insulin action are related to the serum phospholipid fatty acid pattern in healthy men." *Metabolism: Clinical and Experimental,* 1989; 38:188–92.

Rose, D. P., and M. A. Hatala. "Dietary fatty acids and breast cancer: invasion and metastasis." *Nutrition and Cancer,* 1994; 21:103–11.

Schlomo, Y., and R. L. Carasso. "Modulation of learning, pain thresholds, and thermoregulation in the rat by preparations of free purified alpha-linolenic and linoleic acids: determination of the optimal w3-to-w6 ratio." *Proceedings of the National Academy of Sciences,* 1993; 90:10,345–47.

Sears, B. "Essential fatty acids and dietary endocrinology." *Journal of Advanced Medicine,* 1993; 6:211–24.

Sears, B., and B. Lawren. *Enter the Zone.* New York: HarperCollins Publishers, 1995.

Smith, C. J., et al. "Pharmacological analysis of cyclooxygenase-1 in inflammation." *Proceedings of the National Academy of Sciences, USA,* October 27, 1998; 95(22): 13,313–18.

Simopoulos, A. P. "Omega-3 fatty acids in health and disease and in growth and development." *American Journal of Clinical Nutrition,* 1991; 54:438–63.

Willis, A. L. *Handbook of Eicosanoids, Prostaglandins and Related Lipids.* Boca Raton, FL: CRC Press, 1987.

3. NSAIDs and the COX Connection

Alaaedine, N., et al. "Inhibition of tumor necrosis factor alpha-induced prostaglandin E2 production by the anti-inflammatory cytokines interleukin-4, interleukin-10, and interleukin-13 in synovial fibroblasts: distinct targeting in the signaling pathways." *Arthritis and Rheumatism,* April 1999; 42(4):710–18.

Backon, J. "Ginger: inhibition of thromboxane synthetase and stimulation of prostacyclin: relevance for medicine and psychiatry." *Medical Hypotheses,* July 1986; 20(3): 271–78.

Bjorkman, D. J. "The effect of aspirin and nonsteroidal anti-inflammatory drugs on prostaglandins." *American Journal of Medicine,* July 27, 1998; 105(b):8S–12S.

Burton, T. M., and R. Langreth. "Initial Sales Surge for Monsanto Arthritis Drug." *The Wall Street Journal,* January 27, 1999.

Cryer, B., et al. "Cyclooxygenase-1 and cyclooxygenase-2 selectivity of widely used nonsteroidal anti-inflammatory drugs." *American Journal of Medicine,* May 1998; 104(5):413–21.

G. D. Searle and Company. Press release on Celebrex. November 12, 1998.

Geis, G. S. "Update on clinical developments with celecoxib, a new specific COX-2 inhibitor: what can we expect?" *Journal of Rheumatology,* April 1999; 26 Suppl 56: 31–36.

Fort, J. "Celecoxib, a COX-2-specific inhibitor: the clinical data." *American Journal of Orthopedics,* March 1999; 28(3 Suppl):8–12.

Fosslien, E. "Adverse effects of nonsteroidal anti-inflammatory drugs on the gastrointestinal system." *Annals of Clinical Laboratory Science,* March/April 1998; 28(2): 67–81.

Fretland, D. J. "Pharmacological activity of the second generation leukotriene B4 receptor antagonist, SC-53228: effects on colonic inflammation and hepatic function in rodents." *Inflammation,* October 1995; 19(5): 503–15.

Lipsky, P. E. "Specific COX-2 inhibitors in arthritis, oncology, and beyond: where is the science headed?" *Journal of Rheumatology,* April 1999; 26 Suppl 56:25–30.

McAdam, B. F., et al. "Systemic biosynthesis of prostacyclin by cyclooxygenase (COX)-2: the human pharmacology of a selective inhibitor of COX-2." Proceedings of the National Academy of Sciences, January 5, 1999; 96: 272–77.

McIlwain, H. H., and D. F. Bruce. *The Super Aspirin Cure for Arthritis.* New York: Bantam Books, 1999.

Manning, A. "Arthritis enzyme linked to diseases." *USA Today,* August 5, 1998.

Marshall, K. W. "Practical implications of cyclooxygenase-

2-specific inhibitors in orthopedics." *American Journal of Orthopedics,* March 1999; 28(3 Suppl):19–21.

Maslinka, D., and M. Gajewski. "Some aspects of the inflammatory process." *Folia Neuropathologica,* 1998; 36(4):199–204.

Oparil, S., and A. Oberman. "Nontraditional cardiovascular risk factors." *American Journal of Medical Science,* March 1999; 317(3):193–207.

Schmassman, A. "Mechanisms of ulcer healing and effects of nonsteroidal anti-inflammatory drugs." *American Journal of Medicine,* March 30, 1998; 104(3A):43S–51S; discussion 79S–80S.

Schuna, A. A. "Update on treatment of rheumatoid arthritis." *Journal of the American Pharmaceutical Association,* November/December 1998; 38(6):728–36.

Seeds, E. A., "Role of lipoxygenase metabolites in platelet-activating-factor and antigen-induced bronchial hyper-responsiveness and eosinophil infiltration." *European Journal of Pharmacology,* December 7, 1995; 293(4): 369–76.

Sharpe, R. "Several Deaths Show a Link to Celebrex." *The Wall Street Journal,* April 20, 1999.

Simon, L. S. "The evolution of arthritis antiinflammatory care: where are we today?" *Journal of Rheumatology,* April 1999; 26 Suppl 56:11–17.

Simon, L. S., et al. "Preliminary study of safety and efficacy of SC-58635, a novel cyclooxygenase-2 inhibitor." *Arthritis and Rheumatism,* 1998; 41:1591–1602.

Tenenbaum, J. "The epidemiology of nonsteroidal anti-inflammatory drugs." *Canadian Journal of Gastroenterology.* March 1999; 13(2):119–22.

Vane, J. R., et al. "Cyclooxygenases 1 and 2." *Annual Review of Pharmacology Toxicology,* 1998; 38:97–120.

Versteeg, H. H., et al. "Cyclooxygenase-dependent signalling: molecular events and consequences." *FEBS Letter,* February 19, 1999; 445(1):1–5.

Wolfe, S. M., and L. Sasich. "Before the FDA's arthritis drugs advisory committee on the nonsteroidal anti-inflammatory drug (NSAID) Celecoxib (Celebrex)." Statement given on behalf of the Public Citizen's Health Research Group, December 1, 1998.

4. Ginger's Rich Tradition

Fulder, S. *The Ginger Book.* Garden City Park, NY: Avery Publishing Group, 1996.

Govindarajan, V. S. "Ginger—Chemistry, Technology, and Quality Evaluation." *CRC Critical Reviews of Food Sciences and Nutrition,* 1982; 17:1–258.

Mascob, N., et al. "Ethnopharmacological investigations on ginger (Zingiber officinale)." *Journal of Ethnopharmacology,* 1989; 27:129–40.

Sakamura, F. "Changes in volatile constituents of Zingiber officinale during storage." *Phytochemistry,* 1987; 26: 2207–12.

Schulick, P. *Ginger: Common Spice and Wonder Drug,* Third Edition. Brattleboro, VT: Herbal Free Press, Ltd., 1996.

5. Nature's Anti-Inflammatory

Ahmed, R. S., and S. B. Sharma. "Biochemical studies on combined effects of garlic (Allium sativum Linn) and ginger (Zingiber officinale Rosc) in albino rats." *Indian Journal of Experimental Biology,* August 1997; 35(8):841–43.

Amin, A. R., and S. B. Abramson. "The role of nitric oxide in articular cartilage breakdown in osteoarthritis." *Current Opinion in Rheumatology,* May 10, 1998; 263–68.

Attur, M. G., et al. "Autocrine production of IL-1 B by human osteoarthritis-affected cartilage and differential regulation of endogenous nitric oxide, IL-6, prostaglandin E_2 and IL-8." *Proceedings of the Association of American Physicians,* January/February 1998; 110:1, 65–72.

Backon, J. "Mechanism of analgesic effect of clonidine in the treatment of dysmenorrhea." *Medical Hypotheses,* November 1991; 36(3):223–24.

Bhandari, U., N. Sharma, and R. Zafar. "The protective action of ethanolic ginger (Zingiber officinale) extract in cholesterol fed rabbits." *Journal of Ethnopharmacology,* June 1998; 61(2):167–71.

Bordia, A., S. K. Verma, and K. C. Srivastava. "Effect of ginger (Zingiber officinale Rosc.) and fenugreek (Trigonella foenumgraecum L.) on blood lipids, blood sugar and platelet aggregation in patients with coronary artery disease." *Prostaglandins, Leukotrienes, Essential Fatty Acids,* May 1997; 56(5):379–84.

Brown, D., A. Gaby, and R. Reichert. "Clinical applications of natural medicine: Migraine." *Quarterly Review of Natural Medicine,* Summer 1997; 147–58.

Cao, Z. F., et al. "Scavenging effects of ginger on superoxide anion and hydroxyl radical." *Chung Kuo Chung Yoa Tsa Chih,* December 1993; 18(12):750–51, 764.

Fischer, S. M. "Prostaglandins and Cancer." *Frontiers in Bioscience 2,* October 1, 1997; 2:482–500.

Flynn, D., et al. "Inhibition of human neutrophil 5-lipoxygenase activity by gingerdione, shogaol, capsaicin and related pungent compounds." *Prostaglandins, Leukotrienes, and Medicine,* 1986; 24:195–98.

Fries, J. F., et al. "Toward an epidemiology of gastropathy associated with nonsteroidal anti-inflammatory drug use." *Gastroenterology,* 1989; 96:647–55.

Frondosa, C. O., et al. "Expression of pro-inflammatory IL-1 and TNF-alpha by osteoarthritic chondrocytes is altered in response to mechanical stress." Orthopaedic Research Society, 45th Annual Meeting, Anaheim, CA, February 1–4, 1999.

Fulder, S. *The Ginger Book.* Garden City Park, NY: Avery Publishing Group, 1996.

Hashim, S., et al. "Modulatory effects of essential oils from spices on the formation of DNA adduct by aflatoxin B1 in vitro." *Nutrition and Cancer,* 1994; 21(2):169–75.

Katiyar, S. K., R. Agarwal, and H. Mukhtar. "Inhibition of tumor promotion in SENCAR mouse skin by ethanol extract of Zingiber officinale rhizome." *Cancer Research,* March 1, 1996; 56(5):1023–30.

Lee, E., and Y. J. Surj. "Induction of apoptosis in HL-60 cells by pungent vanilloids, [6]-gingerol and [6]-paradol." *Cancer Letters,* December 25, 1998; 134(2):163–68.

Lumb, A. B. "Effect of dried ginger on human platelet function." *Thrombosis and Haemostasis,* January 1994; 71(1):110–11.

Mukherjee, A., et al. "Predictability of the clinical potency of NSAIDs from the preclinical pharmacodynamics in rats." *Inflammation Research,* 1996; 45:531–40.

Murrell, G. A., et al. "Nitric oxide: an important articular free radical." *Journal of Bone and Joint Surgery of America,* February 1996; 78:2, 265–74.

Mustafa, T., and K. C. Srivastava. "Ginger (Zingiber officinale) in migraine headache." *Journal of Ethnopharmacology,* July 1990; 29(3):267–73.

Onogi, T., et al. "Capsaicin-like effect of (6)-shogaol on substance P-containing primary afferents of rats: a possible mechanism of its analgesic action." *Neuropharmacology,* November 1992; 31(11):1165–69.

Park, K. K., et al. "Inhibitory effects of [6]-gingerol, a major pungent principle of ginger, on phorbol ester-induced inflammation, epidermal ornithine decarboxylase activity and skin tumor promotion in ICR mice." *Cancer Letters,* July 17, 1998; 129(2):139–44.

Schulick, P. *Ginger: Common Spice and Wonder Drug,* Third Edition. Brattleboro, VT: Herbal Free Press, Ltd., 1996.

Srivastava, K. C. "Aqueous extracts of onion, garlic and ginger inhibit platelet aggregation and alter arachidonic acid metabolism." *Biomedica Biochimica Acta,* 1984; 43(8–9):S335–46.

———. "Isolation and effects of some ginger components on platelet aggregation and eicosanoid biosynthesis." *Prostaglandins, Leukotrienes, and Medicine,* December 1986; 2–3:187–98.

Surh, Y. J., E. Lee, and J. M. Lee. "Chemoprotective properties of some pungent ingredients present in red pepper and ginger." *Mutation Research,* June 18, 1998; 402(1–2):259–67.

Verma, S. K., et al. "Effect of ginger on platelet aggregation in man." *Indian Journal of Medical Research,* October 1993; 98:240–42.

Westacott, C. I., et al. "Synovial fluid concentration of five different cytokines in rheumatic diseases." *Annals of Rheumatic Diseases,* September 1990; 676–81.

Woolf, C. J., et al. "Cytokines, nerve growth factor and inflammatory hyperalgesia: the contribution of tumor necrosis factor alpha." *British Journal of Pharmacology,* June 12, 1997; 1:3, 417–24.

6. Ginger for a Healthy Digestive System

al-Yahya, M. A., et al. "Gastroprotective activity of ginger zingiber officinale rosc., in albino rats." *American Journal of Chinese Medicine,* 1989; 17(1–2):51–56.

Arfeen, Z., et al. "A double-blind randomized controlled trial of ginger for the prevention of postoperative nausea and vomiting." *Anaesthesia and Intensive Care,* August 1995; 23(4):449–52.

Backon, J. "Ginger and carbon dioxide as thromboxane synthetase inhibitors: potential utility in treating peptic ulceration." *Gut,* 1987; 28:1323.

Golan, R. *Optimal Wellness.* New York: Ballantine Books, 1996.

Goso, Y., et al. "Effects of traditional herbal medicine of gastric mucin against ethanol-induced gastric injury in rats." *Comparative Biochemistry and Physiology,* 1996; 113C;17–21.

Hasenohrl, R. U., et al. "Anxiolytic-like effect of combined extracts of Zingiber officinale and ginkgo biloba in the elevated plus-maze." *Pharmacology, Biochemistry, and Behavior,* February 1996; 53(2):271–75.

Huang, Q. R., et al. "Anti-5-hydroxytryptamine 3 effect of galanolactone, diterpenoid isolated from ginger." *Chemical Pharmacy Bulletin,* February 1991; 39(2): 397–99.

Mowrey, D. B., and D. E. Clayson. "Motion sickness, ginger, and psychophysics." *Lancet,* March 1982; 20(1): 655–57.

Sharma, S. S., and Y. K. Gupta. "Reversal of cisplatin-induced delay in gastric emptying in rats by ginger (Zingiber officinale)." *Journal of Ethnopharmacology,* August 1998; 62(1):49–55.

Stewart, J. J., et al. "Effects of ginger on motion sickness susceptibility and gastric function." *Pharmacology,* 1991; 24(2):111–20.

Wu, H., et al. "Effect of dry ginger and roasted ginger on experimental gastric ulcers in rats." *Chung Kuo Chung Yao Tsa Chih,* May 1990; 15(5):278–80, 317–18.

Yamahara, J., et al. "The anti-ulcer effect in rats of ginger constituents." *Journal of Ethnopharmacology,* July/August 1988; 23(2–3):299–304.

———. "Cholagogic effect of ginger and its active constituents." *Journal of Ethnopharmacology,* May 1985; 13(2):217–25.

———. "Gastrointestinal motility enhancing effect of ginger and its active constituents." *Chemical and Pharmaceutical Bulletin,* 1990.

———. "Inhibition of cytotoxic drug-induced vomiting in suncus by a ginger constituent." *Journal of Ethnopharmacology,* December 1989; 27(3):353–55.

Yoshikawa, M., et al. "Stomachic principles in ginger. III. An anti-ulcer principle, 6-gingesulfonic acid, and three monoacyldigalactosylglycerols, gingerglycolipids A, B, and C, from Zingiberis Rhizoma originating in Taiwan." *Chemical Pharmacy Bulletin* (Tokyo), June 1994; 42(6):1226–30.

Index